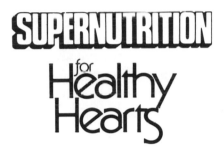

SUPERNUTRITION
for Healthy Hearts

Other books by Richard Passwater

Supernutrition: The Megavitamin Revolution
Guide to Fluorescence Literature,
Volumes 1, 2, and 3

SUPERNUTRITION

for Healthy Hearts

The Total Protection Plan for the
Prevention and Cure of Heart Disease
through Vitamins, Diet, and Exercise

Richard Passwater, Ph. D

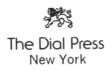

The Dial Press
New York

Chapter 3 was previously published in *Health Quarterly*.

The Dr. Rinse Breakfast is reprinted with permission of *Prevention* magazine. Copyright © 1975 by Rodale Press, Inc. All rights reserved.

Manufactured in the United States of America

First printing

Library of Congress Cataloging in Publication Data

Passwater, Richard A
  Supernutrition for healthy hearts.

  Bibliography: p.
  Includes index.
    1. Heart—Diseases—Prevention. 2. Heart—Diseases—Nutritional aspects. 3. Orthomolecular medicine. I. Title.
  RC682.P37   616.1′2   77-8328
  ISBN O-8037-8035-4

Acknowledgments

It has been a rewarding personal experience to have friends to turn to for answers to questions in their area of expertise or for invigorating discussions. I especially acknowledge the help of the following: Dr. Herb Boynton, Dr. Keith Brewer, Mark Bricklin, Dr. Ray Chen, Dr. Doug Frost, Lee Fryer, Dr. Harold Harper, Ken Halaby, Mort Katz, Dr. Hans Kugler, Wayne Martin, Joe Nowell, Ron Pataki, Jay Patrick, Dr. Linus Pauling, Diane Raintree, Dr. Jacobus Rinse, Dr. Miles Robinson, Jim Scheer, Fred Scott, Ron Sell, Harald Taub, and Bill Wham.

Of course, thanks can never express the blessing of having an understanding wife, who not only tolerates the long hours and messy desk, but also types my manuscripts and adds encouragement.

To Richard and Mike . . .

May heart disease become a rarity in your generation.

And may your hearts always be filled with love and joy, as you have filled our hearts.

Contents

Preface

When a medical breakthrough is first discovered, it's not true. Twenty years later it's true but not important. Thirty years later it's accepted as both true *and* important. But it's fifty years old—we have something better now, and why are you making such a fuss? That's the unnatural history of discoveries in medicine and nutrition, as they are trapped in the aggravated cultural lags which become monuments to unnecessary human suffering.

The opposition of the scientific establishment to innovation is as proverbial as it is irrational. Today women seek the protection of early diagnosis of cancer by the Pap smear, yet its originator published paper after paper for some fifteen years and was ignored. Few know that Fleming was considered to be a little peculiar in his notions about penicillin, and that his discovery preceded the first injection by a gap of years in which the infected unnecessarily died. The electroencephalograph is used today by all neurologists, but it was labeled "electronic quackery" by organized medicine when it was first introduced. Then there's the story of Semmelweis, ridiculed by his medical peers for insisting that they themselves were the vectors for the infections of childbirth. Yet the distrust of discovery remained: The physician who first proposed X-ray treatment for cancer was literally excommunicated by his fellow physicians.

Not only does the establishment in medicine and nutrition stubbornly resist progress, it clings to its mistaken theories with equal tenacity. The low-cholesterol diet, which Richard Passwater exposes for the snare and delusion it is and always has been, *had* to be a fallacious concept, for it was improbable and illogical that the high-cholesterol diet on which man evolved and to which he had obviously adapted could be a non-survival diet. Yet in the name of science millions of people have been persuaded that eggs are lethal, whole milk an invitation to the undertaker, and organ meats—those storehouses of good nutrition—deadly.

As Passwater draws upon his expertise in biochemistry to expose the overlooked evidence that heart disease isn't triggered by the butter on your bread, but may well be touched off by the overprocessing to which the bread itself has been subjected, one is irresistibly tempted to think of the youngster who, with the perceptive eye of childhood, announces that the king is naked. One hopes that those who read this book will promptly realize that the low-cholesterol "solution" to atherosclerosis and cardiac disease is naked, too, devoid of support if one examines, as Passwater does, the scientific literature with the unprejudiced eye of the expert.

We have known for thirty years that Vitamin E is vital to the function of the human heart, that it is a harmless, natural, anti-clotting agent, that it is a valuable (and neglected) aid in cardiac therapy. What we now call "megavitamin" therapy and what many consider as a proposal of recent origin and untested value was actually successfully and harmlessly used in the treatment of arthritis more than thirty years ago. In fact, supernutrition such as Richard Passwater proposes was tested in research at Columbia University before World War II and offered as a means of prolonging the useful lifespan. Not only is Passwater to be commended for his efforts to shorten that lag, but his readers should remember that those who toil to that end, like all pioneers, often pay a price. They are bruised in their efforts to overcome the inertia of the scientific establishment and the apathy of the public. They risk scientific excommunication by their peers who are dedicated to the perpetuation of the status quo—which, in nutrition, is Latin for the strange diet most Americans eat, and for the subnormal health, the disease, and the shortened life expectancy which are among its tolls.

Those who would educate the public in nutrition must have courage to resist the pressures for conformity; must have super-human patience; must be dedicated, determined, and, of course, qualified. Richard Passwater, as those of us who teach avant-garde nutrition well know, is singularly equipped to meet these challenges. As a well-qualified biochemist, he brings to his readers expert, clear guidance in the application of the principles of superior nutrition for superior health. If his readers are wise enough to take full advantage of his expertise, they can convert mere existing into fruitful living, disease into well-being, and passable health into buoyant health.

The actuaries tell us that about sixty percent of you who will read this book will live to be at least sixty-five, but sixty percent of the survivors—one in every three of you reading these lines—will at that age have diabetes, cancer, heart disease, atherosclerosis, or hypertension as your debilitating companion on your way to oblivion. Richard Passwater outlines simple, effective changes in your dietary habits and lifestyle which can negate those statistical probabilities.

There are very few books in which virtually every page carries a truth which may alter the reader's destiny for the better. This is such a book, and those who study it and apply its nutritional truths will come to understand, gratefully, why we in the field of nutrition deeply appreciate the scientists who, like Passwater, are willing to come out of the laboratory to address (and help) the medical profession and the public.

Carlton Fredericks, Ph.D., F.I.A.P.M.

Foreword

Supernutrition for Healthy Hearts is a landmark in nutritional therapy. It is a carefully annotated, thorough, balanced, and readable nutritional handbook.

Richard Passwater has done his homework well. He has selected and offers exciting scientific evidence that there is scientific salvation for those who are heart attack prone. He has not succumbed to the pressure of the usual commercial influences that prevail in many research projects. His instructions present the details of a nutritional feast for sick cells that have been starved for the essential nutrients.

Here is a bonanza of helpful nutritional information that can make the difference between having a heart attack and not having one. Your application of these principles—or your lack of applying them—may determine the quality of your health and the length of your life.

Richard Passwater is an unusual researcher in that he does not belittle or disdain the clinical observations and experiences of those physicians who have added much to medicine with their data. He seems to be one of the few scientific researchers who realizes that the major advances in the progress of medicine have been made by astute clinical observers.

It has been my privilege to have observed for the past twenty-five years the clinical benefits of most of the measures explained so well in this book. I have seen the clinical value of nutritional therapy being added to the usual medical therapeutic measures. I have given large doses of vitamin C intravenously for more than thirty years usually with beneficial results. Some results have been outstanding.

It has been rewarding that as a pioneer in the field of

preventive medicine I have been actively engaged in monitoring and measuring blood sugar levels since 1950. My patients know that the therapeutic augmentation of concentrated nutrients is very beneficial.

It is extremely fortunate that the focus of this book is on the prevention of heart attacks rather than on the extreme dramatic measures that are needed when the heart attack actually occurs. This approach can result in billions of dollars in savings for the sick care of the American people.

Supernutrition for Healthy Hearts is an invaluable guide to better health, less worry, and lower medical costs. It is completely unpretentious and written honestly for real, down-to-earth human beings who treasure their health and happiness.

Dr. Richard O. Brennan
Chairman, Board of Trustees, International Academy of
Preventive Medicine
Author, *Nutrigenetics*

Introduction

The compelling need to write *Supernutrition for Healthy Hearts* became evident after I had many conversations with and received many letters from readers following the publication of my earlier book, *Supernutrition: Megavitamin Revolution.* It was surprising to learn that not only general readers, but also physicians, were not informed of the recent research proving that dietary cholesterol was not a factor in heart disease.

I expected to find confusion about blood cholesterol levels and heart disease, but what I discovered was that definitive tests from around the world, including the often misquoted Framingham study which eventually exonerated dietary cholesterol, had not been presented in popular health literature.

As long as we are misled as to the true cause of heart disease, we cannot take the proper steps to prevent it—nor can our doctors. The fear of cholesterol (cholesterolphobia) caused by this misinformation often conditions people to eat unbalanced diets by avoiding eggs, whole milk, butter, and meat. The resulting dietary deficiencies can actually cause premature heart disease.

Another compounding factor is the erroneous belief that polyunsaturates can prevent or cure heart disease. Many people are consuming potentially harmful amounts of polyunsaturates in a misguided effort to prevent heart disease.

The cholesterol and polyunsaturates theories of heart disease are nice and simple, but have been disproven. The explanation is presented in Chapters 3 through 8 of this book. The failure of this information to reach outside the laboratories and clinics of the immediate researchers involved has motivated me to expand upon my discussion of heart disease in *Supernutrition: Megavitamin Revolution,* and fully describe the results of the latest research into the cause of heart disease.

I felt it was important to elaborate on the recently determined real cause of heart disease: monoclonal proliferation. Monoclonal proliferation was postulated as a cause of heart disease by Dr. Earl Benditt of the University of Washington, and I have expanded his observations with the results of my own research involving "free radical pathology." These theories and terms are explained simply in a non-technical fashion. Only by understanding the cause of heart disease can we know what to do to prevent it from striking us prematurely.

I also felt the need to bring to the general public successful programs of heart-disease therapy such as Dr. Rinse's Breakfast, which has benefitted more than 10,000 people who had been suffering from **mild** coronary disease.

By combining the methods developed by Dr. Rinse, myself, and others, I have developed a total protection plan for the avoidance of premature heart disease through vitamins, diet, and exercise. The plan is simple as A . . . B . . . C . . . D . . . E . . . F. Six steps encourage you to eat good food and enjoy life in essentially your present lifestyle. The steps involve Antioxidant vitamins (primarily C and E), Blood pressure control, Cigarette smoking reduction, Diet control (total caloric intake), mild Exercise and replacing as much frustration as possible with Fun.

This program will reverse plaque formation to open up your arteries, improve your blood circulation, put more available oxygen in your bloodstream, strengthen your heart, and improve your heart energy. In about three months your heart can be five years younger than it is today and, in another six months your heart can be ten or more years younger than it was when you began the program.

It is my hope that if the fallacies of the cholesterol theory are brought to the attention of physicians and the general public alike, premature heart disease could be reduced by sixty to eighty percent of the present national rate. This book cannot guarantee total protection to everyone, since factors such as genetics and perhaps some factors which remain to be discovered are involved in heart disease. But I definitely feel, based on projections of studies I conducted, that about eighty percent of those prone to premature coronary thrombosis can be protected.

I hope the information that I have brought together will benefit those readers already having heart disease. Even if you have severe heart disease, it is possible to return to a healthful life. Some heart attack victims have been thankful that their attack served as a warning to improve their nutrition and lifestyle, and now they feel better than in many years.

I wish to introduce to those with advanced heart disease a little known but very encouraging treatment—chelation therapy. Over the past twenty-five years, thousands who have been judged to be inoperable have chosen this lifesaving option and returned to active lives. The length and health of your life is very much a matter of how well you care for yourself. You can save your own life.

I hope that readers will also accept the responsibility to learn cardiopulmonary resuscitation, a technique introduced in the appendices, so that they can save a heart attack victim if the need arises.

I have felt a responsibility to offer the soundest information now available concerning the prevention and alleviation of heart disease. It is your responsibility to consider the evidence and adjust your lifestyle to these principles of heart health as best you can.

Superhealth to you all.

Richard Passwater
Silver Spring, Maryland
1977

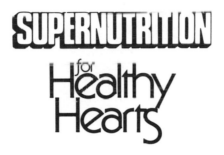

SUPERNUTRITION
for Healthy Hearts

Total Protection against Heart Disease Is Now Possible

Only in 1974 was the actual cause of heart disease, America's leading cause of premature death, determined. A little more than a year later, the studies pinpointing the cause were confirmed.

Many will be surprised to hear that dietary cholesterol was not found to be the culprit. It is now believed, as a result of the studies by Dr. Earl P. Benditt (of the University of Washington School of Medicine, Seattle), that the cholesterol found in the arteries at the site of the plaques (deposits) that cause heart disease is an end product of the cellular deterioration that produced the narrowed arteries (called atherosclerosis), not the cause.

The majority of recent books on the prevention of heart disease promote the avoidance of cholesterol. Yet, no matter how carefully you follow the low-cholesterol diets, no matter how many eggs or pats of butter or glasses of milk you have dropped from your diet, you still have a 50 percent chance of dying prematurely from a heart attack. The reason for this bad news is simply that cholesterol is not the cause of heart disease.

For the benefit of those led to believe that dietary cholesterol and fats are the culprits and polyunsaturated fats are the cures, dramatic evidence is presented in Chapters 4 through 8 to prove that you have been misled.

Fortunately, now that its cause is understood, total protection against heart disease is possible. The essentials of that protection are a balanced diet, regular exercise, control of blood pressure, cigarette smoking, and stress, plus daily vitamin and mineral supplements rich in antioxidant nutrients. Chief among the supplements are the antioxidant vitamins E and C, and in strong supporting roles are the lesser-known nutrients (generally lacking in American diets) pangamate (vitamin B_{15}) and the antioxidant trace mineral selenium.

The Supernutrition Program (p. 301) indicates how much of these supplements you need and how often you should take them. The program is designed to fit individual needs. The amount of supplements you take is based on your own health as indicated by your answers to the Supernutrition Quiz (p. 289). Individual chapters that precede the program explain why exercise; the control of blood pressure, cigarettes, diet, and stress; plus particular vitamin and mineral supplements are suggested for total protection against heart disease. The Total Protection Plan is outlined at the end of this chapter (p. 7), and a chart to help you monitor your progress toward total protection is presented in the final chapter (p. 279).

By following the Total Protection Plan, it is possible to make your heart five years younger in three months, and ten years younger in nine months. Even if you presently have heart disease, those improvements are possible.

For those with moderate heart disease, a daily supplement of "heart foods"—Dr. Rinse's Breakfast (p. 266)—is suggested as part of the Total Protection Plan.

For those with severe heart disease, chelation therapy (p. 248), a safe and relatively inexpensive nonsurgical technique for freeing your arteries of deposits, can save your life. This little-known therapy, currently practiced by about one thousand American doctors, makes the risky and costly coronary-bypass operation unnecessary.

Once your arteries have been freed of deposits, either with Dr. Rinse's Breakfast or by chelation therapy, the Total Protection Plan can insure you that your heart will remain in the best of health.

Hopefully, now that the cause of arterial plaque formation is understood, the American diet will include fewer highly refined and processed foods with harmful artificial additives, and larger (and more healthful) quantities of eggs, milk, and butter.

The Mistakes That Led to the Cholesterol Scare

One of the mistakes made by many heart-disease researchers in attempting to understand the cause of heart disease has been in examining the suspected heart-disease risk factors as independent variables in a cause-and-effect relationship. That may sound complicated, but it isn't.

By holding all factors in an experiment constant except the one being tested, and then varying only that factor, researchers have attempted to correlate the results of their experiments with the variation of the factor being tested. The problem is that this standard type of research has not sufficiently explained the causes of heart disease, and for good reason

To get heart disease, one does not have to seriously overdo one of the real risk factors; that is, sedentary lifestyle, unbalanced nutrition, high blood pressure, smoking, immoderate stress, or calorie imbalance. In fact, many who do seriously overdo one factor (and only one factor) don't get heart disease at all. Overdoing alone can be compensated for by a healthy body, or can lead to a mild form of heart disease free of clinical symptoms or problems.

But, invariably when two or more real risk factors are slightly abused, heart disease will occur. And the abuses may be so slight as to be considered normal living. For example, you can avoid exercise completely, yet follow all other heart-health guidelines to the hilt and not develop premature heart disease. But if your diet is less than perfect and you don't exercise quite enough, then it's no longer a question of whether you will get heart disease, but how seriously and when. And this is the case for most Americans.

We can survive atherosclerosis (the deposits in the arteries that lead to narrowed arteries and increased risk of clot formation) if our blood remains slippery (as a result of a sound nutrition) or if we increase' artery diameter (as a result of exercise). But if we have arteries narrowed by deposits and sticky blood, then heart disease becomes fatal.

Most Americans have been just a little too casual in too many areas of heart-disease risk. We haven't been seriously overdoing any one risk factor and we feel that being a little lax here and there won't hurt. After all, we have cut back on eggs and butter, added a pat of margarine, and usually exercise a little every day and more on the weekends. The good news is that we need only slight changes to achieve total protection against heart disease.

The bad news is that too many people have cholesterol-phobia (the needless and unfounded fear of dietary cholesterol) and their nutrition has suffered because of it. They believe that a pat of margarine and an egg substitute will protect them from heart disease. This belief detracts from a realistic approach to the prevention of heart disease. It is not the public's fault. Many are doing their best. But they have been misled. Chapters 4 through 8 will open their eyes.

Originally physicians and scientists viewed the cholesterol deposits that accumulate in arteries as being caused by too much cholesterol in the blood. And many went even further to reason that the excess blood cholesterol came from eating too much cholesterol in our food. Even though the famous Framingham study proved this notion wrong in 1970, the myth has continued to have popular support. A few tests in the late 1950s and early 1960s at first appeared to confirm the apparent obviousness of the cholesterol-cause theory. Then better-controlled and properly conducted experiments in the late 1960s and early 1970s disproved both links to heart disease.

Each of the following studies has shown that low-cholesterol diets don't reduce heart disease:

- The St. Mary's Hospital Trial (1965)
- The London research committee Trial (1965)

- The Norwegian Trial (1966)
- The Anti-Coronary Club Trial (1966)
- The London Medical Research Council Trial (1968)
- The National Diet Heart Study (1968)
- The Finnish Mental Hospital Trial (1968)
- The Los Angeles Veterans' Trial (1969)
- The Framingham Study (1970)
- The Ireland-Boston Heart Study (1970)
- The St. Vincent's Hospital Trial (1973)
- The Diet and Coronary Heart Disease Study in England (1974)
- The Edinburgh-Stockholm Study (1975)
- The Minnesota Study (1975)
- The UCLA Study (1975)
- The Honolulu-Japanese Study (1975)
- Additionally, the Coronary Drug Project in 1974 showed that drugs that reduced blood cholesterol were of no value in preventing heart disease.

Yet we hear little of these studies.

It is now known that the arterial deposits that cause heart disease don't form as a result of high blood cholesterol levels and that eating more cholesterol doesn't raise the amount of cholesterol in your blood. The proof that high-cholesterol diets don't cause heart disease is in Chapters 4 and 5, and the proof that low-cholesterol diets don't prevent heart disease is in Chapters 6 through 8.

The Real Cause of Heart Disease

Newer research has shown that the deposits form because of cell proliferation in the artery walls (similar to the cellular growth of cancer).

The research that fully explains plaque formation in the arteries was conducted from 1970 to 1974 by Dr. Earl P. Benditt and his colleagues at the University of Washington School of Medicine (specifics were published in the *American Journal of Pathology* in 1974). This research was confirmed by Dr. Robert Heptinstall of the Johns Hopkins School of Medicine in 1975 (results published in the *American Journal of Pathology*, 1975).

In the course of his studies, Dr. Benditt discovered that the cells in the artery wall proliferate because of mutation in their DNA (reproduction mechanism) caused by cigarette-smoke chemicals, free radicals (highly reactive molecular fragments), low-level radiation, epoxides (normal metabolic breakdown products) of fatty substances, chlorine, and other chemical mutagens circulating in the bloodstream, as well as chemicals released by the arteries as a result of high blood pressure.

The proliferating cells form lesions that vary in color from faint yellowish-gray to a pearl-gray. Sophisticated analytical techniques have revealed that the lesions' major constituents are collagen (a connective-tissue protein) and glycosaminoglycans (a carbohydrate–amino-acid complex) embedded in a matrix of smooth muscle cells. Cholesterol and other fats are produced from within the lesion cells (all cells can make cholesterol). Excess cholesterol production is stimulated because of the physical pressure exerted on these lesion cells as they are squeezed against the normal artery tissue.

Therefore, the old belief that the deposits in the arteries are principally caused by cholesterol does not hold up to the newer sophisticated electron-microscope techniques using advanced selective staining procedures, which show that cholesterol appears only after the lesion has formed.

No wonder blood cholesterol and dietary cholesterol levels do not affect heart disease (and no study to date has been able to prove that they do)—cholesterol is not the initial plaque material, but merely a by-product of disintegrating cells that have proliferated. Some cholesterol is attracted from the bloodstream to the artery by an electronic charge in the final stage of plaque formation, but this process is also independent of blood cholesterol level or dietary cholesterol intake. (Even if blood cholesterol levels were so low as to threaten the life of the individual—and that is possible although unlikely—cholesterol would still be extracted from the bloodstream by the artery at that point.)

The process of plaque formation will be explained in detail in Chapter 3 and the experiments that encouraged the development of the Total Protection Plan will be explained throughout the rest of the book.

The Total Protection Plan

Total protection against heart disease is as simple as A, B, C. Actually, since protection involves a six-point program, it's as simple as A, B, C . . . D, E, F. The plan is easy to remember, because It's:

- A for Antioxidant Nutrients
- B for Blood Pressure
- C for Cigarettes (Reduce)
- D for Diet
- E for Exercise
- and F for Fun (not Frustration)

The Total Protection Plan doesn't necessarily require that you give up smoking entirely or have ideal weight. It does require that you follow the guidelines. None of the six protective factors is beyond your ability. All are important.

Chapter 32 personalizes the Total Protection Plan by explaining the step-by-step details of the Supernutrition Program through which you can determine the level of vitamin and mineral supplements you need, and by providing a Total Protection Plan chart to help you monitor your progress in controlling blood pressure, cigarette smoking, diet, exercise level, and frustration.

The following chapters will answer the important questions about heart disease that concern you. Subjects discussed include the following:

Essential Topics for Those Free of Heart Disease and for Those Who Want to Be

- What has caused several skeptics of vitamin E to change their minds.

- How taking vitamin C and the minerals magnesium and chromium will help protect you from heart disease.
- Why vitamin B₁₅ should be on the dining table of all persons over forty years of age.
- Why women are increasingly entering the heart-disease statistics. Twenty years ago, according to one study, men had twelve times the rate of heart disease of women. Now it's down to four times their rate.
- What effects birth-control pills have had on the rising rate of heart disease in women.
- Why only ten pounds of excess body weight after the age of forty-five decreases your life span by 8 percent.
- How to keep calories down and weight off.
- Why large meals can bring on heart attacks and why we should eat several small meals instead.
- How to stop smoking without gaining weight.
- How heart attacks can be predicted. How your ears can indicate hardening of the arteries.
- What exercise can do and what it cannot do.
- Exercising to prevent heart disease.
- What effect Type A personality has on heart disease. Various stresses and how they affect you. How to overcome stress.
- How excess polyunsaturated fats can harm you.
- Why the 1970 Kannel report of the Framingham study showing no relationship between food cholesterol content and heart-disease incidence has been ignored.
- What you should know about new research on the minerals selenium and zinc.
- How soft water makes your arteries hard.
- How chlorine kills germs in your water but damages your arteries. What can be done?
- The effect that fiber and sugar in your diet have on heart disease.
- Why the incidence of high blood pressure is on the increase. How mind-over-matter can lower high blood pressure.

Essential Topics for Those with Heart Disease

- Dangerous combinations of heart-disease drugs that could ruin your sex drive or even kill you.

- Heart drugs that may cause cancer.
- The drugs that lowered blood-cholesterol levels yet caused 40 percent more heart-attack deaths.
- Exercising to recuperate from heart disease.
- Sex after the coronary.
- How a daily regimen of special "heart food" supplements— Dr. Rinse's Breakfast—can cure those with moderate heart disease.
- How chelation therapy frees clogged arteries of deposits quickly, safely, and painlessly (and makes the risky and expensive arterial-bypass operation unnecessary) for those with advanced heart disease.

The Number-One Killer

Heart disease (all types of cardiovascular disease—that is, coronary thrombosis, calcified valves, and congenital defects) is our number-one killer in this country, striking down approximately a million Americans each year. Heart attack (coronary thrombosis) alone kills nearly 700,000 Americans annually, mostly men. Coronary thrombosis must be considered epidemic, since no case of it was known before 1890. Between 1900 and 1965, the coronary epidemic struck down younger men in each succeeding decade.

Statistical evidence shows that the epidemic is slightly receding as the deaths from coronary thrombosis in younger men have recently decreased. Numerous studies suggest that the improvement is not a result of following low-cholesterol diets. Most likely this decrease is due to better nutritional habits (including health foods and vitamins), increased physical activity, reduction in smoking, and better emergency care.

Formerly many potential heart-disease risk factors were proposed. Now the real risk factors have been pinpointed (see Chapter 3), and total protection against heart disease is possible. Today it is easy to beat the odds of getting heart disease.

2
An Epidemic Has Hit Us

Coronary thrombosis is truly a product of modern lifestyles —therefore, many believe that a change in lifestyle back to the "good ole days" is all that's required to prevent it. While that would certainly help, our food and environment are not what they were in the good ole days; and both are factors in the heart-disease epidemic.

Yet many people have not accepted the epidemic nature of heart disease, believing that heart disease has always been with us and is simply more prevalent now because people are living longer. They point out that the average lifespan, which is now nearing 72 years, was only 47.3 years in 1900. Since heart disease doesn't normally occur until after 50 years of age, those who fail to recognize the heart-disease epidemic further reason that since there were few people living long enough to get heart disease in the nineteenth century, physicians simply didn't pay much attention to it.

Let's examine the premise that people didn't live long enough to get heart disease in the nineteenth century. It is true that the *average* lifespan was 47.3 years in 1900, but that figure is misleading in that it was disproportionately lowered by the large number of infant and childhood deaths. Nowadays better sanitation and antibiotics have helped cut infectious diseases, which formerly caused many deaths among young mothers after delivery, infants, and young children. For a better indication of the life expectancy of the adult population, let's look at the lifespan remaining for those reaching 20 years of age then and today. There hasn't been much change. The belief that adults are living significantly longer today is false.

As an example, those reaching their twentieth birthday in 1900 could, on an average, expect to live until they were 62.2. In 1920, those reaching 20 years could expect to survive until they were 65.6 years old. In 1940, those reaching 20 lived on the average to 67.8 years, and in 1960 the average 20-year-old could reasonably hope to reach 70.3. These figures reveal an increase of only 8 years in life expectancy for adults between 1900 and 1960. Similarly, there has been little change in the life expectancy of those reaching 65 years of age then and now. The average remaining years for those reaching 65 years of age was 11.5 years in 1900 and 12.9 in 1960: an increase of only 1.4 years since 1900. In fact, the average age of the population was older in the early 1900s than it was in the 1960s and is today. The percentage of the population over 30 years of age was 56.9 in 1940, 55.7 in 1960, and 54.1 in 1970.

Coronary Thrombosis—The Twentieth-Century Disease

When you compare the deaths from heart diseases such as calcified valves, rheumatic heart, and other congenital heart defects per 100,000 population in the 1900s to those of today, there's not much difference. Yet the death rate from coronary thrombosis (a clot blocking the flow of blood to heart) has climbed from 0 (no recorded cases) in 1890 to nearly 340 deaths per 100,000 people in 1970. In 1914 the four most common forms of heart disease were rheumatic (46.3 percent), hypertensive (19.5 percent), enlargement (15.5 percent), and syphilitic (12.3 percent). (Dr. R. C. Cabot, *Journal of the American Medical Association,* 1914.) In the 1930s, the four most prevalent forms were hypertensive, coronary, rheumatic, and syphilitic heart disease, in that order. (Dr. P. D. White, *Bulletin of the New York Academy of Medicine,* 1940.) Now coronary heart disease ranks first due to the epidemic nature of coronary thrombosis. Table 2.1 reveals the alarming increase of the disease during the decades of the 1950s and 1960s.

Table 2.1

Death Rates, 1950–1970 (per 100,000 U.S. population)

	Coronary Heart Disease	All Heart Diseases	All Causes of Death
1950	213.0	356.8	963.8
1951	219.6	357.0	966.7
1952	226.2	357.6	961.4
1953	236.1	361.3	959.0
1954	235.7	348.3	919.0
1955	247.0	356.5	930.4
1956	255.5	361.0	935.1
1957	265.6	369.4	958.6
1958	266.2	367.7	950.8
1959	268.6	363.2	938.6
1960	275.6	369.0	954.7
1961	274.4	362.4	929.5
1962	283.8	370.1	945.0
1963	289.8	375.2	961.3
1964	285.0	365.7	939.6
1965	288.6	367.4	943.2
1966	292.7	371.2	951.3
1967	288.7	364.5	935.7
1968	337.6	372.6	965.7
1969	331.7	366.1	951.9
1970	340.0	377.6	945.3

Data from USDHEW.

What is especially disconcerting, beyond the high number of deaths, is the number of people dying *prematurely* from this new form of heart disease. And it definitely is a new form. Some of the best surgeons and pathologists in history were studying causes of death in the last half of the nineteenth century, and yet coronary thrombosis was not discovered until 1896.

A few researchers believe that coronaries in earlier centuries could have been diagnosed as "apoplexy" (sudden stroke), but the symptoms and obvious expiration signs of apoplexy are grossly different from those of coronaries. Few physicians would mistake one for the other. Besides, the deaths per 100,000 population due to apoplexy were much less than would be required to hide our coronary epidemic.

The symptoms of a heart attack—severe chest pressure, chest and arm pain, cold sweats, nausea, fall in blood pressure, rapid weak pulse, etc.—are so dramatic that few doctors could have missed recognizing heart attacks, even if they had occurred at merely one-thousandth the rate of today. In 1930 it took a specialist to identify a coronary because of its rarity; today, heart attack is so common the average person can spot it from a distance. In 1940 coronary thrombosis was an old man's disease; today approximately 200,000 persons *under 65 years of age* die each year of it. It even strikes down some women as young as 20.

Evidence based on the autopsies of mummies reveals that deposits in the arteries (atherosclerosis) were common in the days of ancient Egypt. Yet, there are no signs that in those days the blood formed clots in the narrowed arteries to cause thrombosis or an infarct (an area of dead tissue caused by loss of blood supply). One 2,100-year-old mummy from Changsha, China, revealed that an individual had an arterial disease but had not experienced a heart attack, which is certainly possible. Adequate antioxidants, which at that time could have come from whole grains In the diet, and/or activity could have prevented the blood from clotting in the slightly narrowed arteries. Atheromatous arteries (those having plaque) were reported before coronaries were discovered. And so was cholesterol. Cholesterol was found in plaque in 1843 by Dr. J. Vogel several decades after the sugar beet was introduced to Europe by Napoleon in 1815. (Voss, Leipzig, 1843)

The case linking heart disease to modern lifestyle—physical inactivity and poor diet (both food selection and food quality)—is strengthened by comparing general adult health during different time periods. According to anthropologist Dr. Robert McCracken of Denver, Colorado, if you were to set the average caveman against today's average man, there's little doubt the caveman would win every type of physical competition. In a 1975 Denver lecture, Dr. McCracken said that diet is the main reason twentieth-century man is in such poor condition: "Man is supposed to eat meat, vegetables, and fruit. Instead he's eating a lot of stuff he's not designed to—and it's killing him." Dr. McCracken questions whether man's health has improved at all: "All the medical gadgets and research of the last 10,000 years have added up to zero when it comes to the general health advancements in the world."

Dr. Lawrence Power (of Wayne State University and Chief of Medicine at Detroit General Hospital) estimates that 20 percent of otherwise healthy American men develop heart-disease symptoms during their 40s and 50s, and that one-third of these will die prematurely as a result. According to Dr. Power, "Our civilization, our way of life, exposes us to greater risk of a heart attack. Among other things, we are the first culture in history to derive half our calories from processed food. More and more people are having heart attacks in their twenties. We are living in an epidemic of coronary heart disease."

Dr. Paul Dudley White, one of the first and most famous American cardiologists, often spoke of the epidemic nature of coronary thrombosis. In an article by Maria Wilhelm, Dr. White stated: "First of all, I want to emphasize that heart disease truly is an epidemic today, a fact that many people seem to refuse to accept. . . . Your generation has become so used to the specter of heart attacks, you don't even conceive of life free from this danger. But remember, when I was an intern at Massachusetts General Hospital in 1911, there was no Department of Cardiology." (*Family Circle,* 1971)

Coronary thrombosis was first reported in 1896 by Dr. George Dock, as he attested in a later report (*Journal of the American Medical Association,* 1939). Yet the disease was still an obscure medical curiosity in 1912 when Chicago physician Dr. J. B. Herrick discussed six cases in the *Journal of the American Medical Association.*

And when Dr. White set up the first cardiology laboratory

in 1920, coronary thrombosis was still so uncommon that most medical students did not know of the disease until after their formal training. Although Dr. White brought a crude electrocardiograph back from a European trip in 1914, the modern type of electrocardiograph did not appear until 1944. And it was not until the 1950s that physicians began routinely monitoring blood levels of cholesterol because of the steadily increasing death rate from heart disease.

Heart attacks have been our leading cause of death for only the last thirty years. Presently they are killing more than 700,000 people a year (772,570 in 1975)—an astonishing increase from the two or three people that died of heart attack each year in the early 1900s. According to the American Heart Association (AHA), diseases of the heart and blood vessels claim more American lives than all other causes of death combined.

As can be seen in Table 2.2, the annual death rate per 100,000 population has been cut nearly in half since 1900. Diseases such as pneumonia and influenza, acute kidney infection, tuberculosis, appendicitis, and other infectious diseases have dropped to very low levels. Yet in that same period, the annual death rate from heart disease has nearly tripled. (Yet our population is younger today than it was in the early decades of the century.)

Of the 136,231 people who died of heart disease in 1912, only 6 (less than 0.01 percent) were reported to have died from coronary thrombosis, while of the 745,200 people who died from heart disease in 1968, more than 600,000 (that's more than 80 percent) were reported to have died from coronary thrombosis.

The biggest change occurred in 1952, when the death rate from coronary thrombosis was three times the 1950 rate, and 12 times the rate of 1945.

The most discouraging factor in this increase has been the expansion of coronary thrombosis into the younger age groups. During the 1950s and 1960s, nearly each year produced a record quarter of a million deaths from heart disease (virtually all due to coronaries) in the

Table 2.2

Causes of Death, 1900–1971 (per 100,000 U.S. population)

Year	1900	1912	1926	1955	1968	1970	1971
Population (millions)	76.0	95.4	117.1	165.2	200.1	203.2	207.9
Death Rate—All Causes	1,719.1	1,338.8	1,222.7	929.5	965.7	945.3	931.9
Death Rate—Heart Disease (not including stroke)	137.4	142.8	175.8	352.0	372.6	377.6	391.1
Stroke and Related Deaths	106.9	77.5	86.3	106.6	105.8	101.9	100.9
Cancer Death Rate	64.0	77.1	94.9	147.6	159.4	162.8	161.4
Diabetes	11.0	15.0	18.0	15.2	19.2	18.9	18.3
Pneumonia and Influenza	202.2	142.9	143.2	27.5	36.8	30.9	27.3
Appendicitis	?	11.6	15.0	1.0	0.7	?	0.0±
Acute Kidney Infection	?	103.2	98.3	1.4	4.7	?	3.6
Liver Cirrhosis	12.5	13.5	7.2	10.8	14.6	15.5	15.6
Tuberculosis	?	149.7	87.1	9.5	2.6	?	2.1
Other Infectious Diseases	?	131.8	75.2	7.0	6±	?	5.3

Data from USDHEW—HRA, and Bellew and Bellew. The data base for 1900 and 1970 is not exactly the same as for the rest.

younger age groups—usually among men in their 50s and 40s.

Brighter Prospects Today for Younger Men

The heartening news is that though the overall coronary-thrombosis rate continues to climb higher, the death rate in the 35-to-64 age bracket has begun to drop. Nearly 10 percent fewer men 35 to 44 years old died from heart disease in 1973 than had in 1963. During the same years, in the 45-to-54 age group 12.5 percent fewer men died of heart disease, and in the 55-to-64 age group 10.5 percent fewer men died in 1973 than had in 1963. In 1975, the combined deaths from heart disease and strokes fell under the million level (918,200) for the first time since 1967. The epidemic for younger men may have peaked in 1963, as Table 2.3 suggests.

The lowered death rate does not necessarily mean that fewer men are getting heart disease. Exact reasons why fewer young men are dying from heart disease are not known, but they may well include better care during the first minutes of the attack with widespread use of mobile intensive-care units in urban areas, better medication and treatment within the first day of the attack, increased physical activity, improved weight control and better blood-pressure control in a conscious effort to prevent heart disease, plus the use of vitamin E by an estimated 30 million Americans. Additionally, a survey by the National Clearinghouse for Smoking and Health in Atlanta, Georgia, showed that the proportion of male smokers 21 and over dropped from 52.8 percent in 1964 to 39.3 percent in 1975.

Disheartening News for Women

With the exception of the most recent figures (1974), the heart-attack death rate for women in the U.S. has been generally on the increase. Even considering the recent slight

Table 2.3

Coronary Heart-Disease Death Rates by Age Group
(per 100,000 U.S. population in each age group)

	Age Groups					
Year	35–44	45–54	55–64	65–74	75–84	85+
1958	58.0	232.7	658.4	1,628.8	3,364.8	7,069.3
1959	57.6	233.7	655.3	1,643.6	3,359.2	7,321.0
1960	57.7	238.0	665.5	1,553.7	3,434.8	7,296.5
1961	57.9	235.2	649.4	1,541.4	3,360.6	7,383.3
1962	58.7	238.4	660.4	1,586.7	3,449.2	7,922.2
1963	61.0	240.3	668.4	1,619.1	3,495.6	8,165.6
1964	61.0	235.8	660.3	1,586.7	3,388.6	7,885.7
1965	60.0	236.6	657.4	1,584.0	3,422.0	8,088.2
1966	59.6	236.4	661.4	1,609.9	3,413.6	8,037.7
1967	60.1	231.4	645.0	1,568.8	3,334.2	7,941.8
1968	56.9	216.8	624.1	1,552.2	3,441.7	8,496.7
1969	55.4	210.3	598.4	1,500.3	3,367.6	8,400.2
1970	52.9	206.5	585.5	1,429.2	3,406.3	7,249.4
1971	52.1	202.3	574.4	1,385.8	3,356.8	7,780.4
1972	50.2	199.5	569.6	1,383.1	3,371.0	7,712.0
1973	48.3	194.9	559.5	1,333.4	3,322.9	7,692.6

Data from USDHEW.

decline, the increase is drastically above historical levels. According to the AHA, more women died of heart disease than from any other cause in 1974—twice as many as from cancer and accidents combined. The reasons for the increase may be that more women are smoking, holding down stressful jobs, and taking birth-control pills.

Two recent British studies strongly suggest that users of oral contraceptives run a greater risk of developing coronary thrombosis than nonusers. The reports by Dr. Joel Mann (a lecturer in social medicine at Oxford University) and Dr. William Inman (an official of the British Government's Committee on the Safety of Medicines) were published in 1975 in the *British Medical Journal.* Furthermore, it has long been established that birth-control pill users have an increased risk of stroke, blood clots in the lungs (pulmonary embolism), and clots in the leg veins (thrombophlebitis). (Dr. Robert W. Kistner, *Postgraduate in Medicine,* 1964.)

Among middle-aged women using the pill, the risk of death from coronary thrombosis is 3 times greater than among nonusers. According to Dr. Inman, even the risk of nonfatal heart attack in women between 30 and 39 years of age using the pill is 2.7 times that of nonusers.

The relationship between oral contraceptives and high blood pressure in young women was first reported in 1967. In 1974, a report in the *New England Journal of Medicine* revealed that women using the pill are 9 times more likely to develop heart disease than nonusers.

Prior to the slight decrease in 1974, coronary-thrombosis deaths among women had been steadily on the rise. Deaths from coronaries among women under age 45 was 11 percent higher in 1962 to 1968 than in 1955 to 1961. In 1955, men under 51 years of age were 12 times more vulnerable to heart attacks than women of the same age, but in 1967–71, men were only 4 times more vulnerable (Dr. David Spain, *Science News,* 1973).

Cholesterol and Saturated Fats Are Not the Villains

Notice that I did not credit cholesterol reduction or polyunsaturated-fat increase with playing a role in the recent reductions of heart disease.

The amount of saturated fat and cholesterol in the American diet has remained essentially unchanged since 1910. In 1948, the average American ate 4 more grams of saturated fat (primarily animal fats, such as in milk, butter, cheese, beef, pork, poultry, etc.) each day than in 1910. Since it takes 28.4 grams to make an ounce, the increase per day was only one-seventh of an ounce. In 1958, the amount of saturated fat in the average American diet was

Table 2.4

Daily per capita intake of selected nutrients.

Year	Calories	Cholesterol mg.	FAT			CARBOHYDRATE			P/S
			Total (grams)	Animal % (mostly saturates)	Vegetable % (mostly polyunsaturates)	Total (grams)	Starch %	Sucrose %	
1909–1913	3,490	495	125	83.1	17.0	492	68.3	31.7	0.20
1925–1929	3,470	—	135	78.2	21.8	476	58.7	41.3	0.28
1935–1939	3,270	—	133	73.3	26.8	436	56.8	43.2	0.37
1947–1949	3,230	561	141	74.6	25.6	403	52.4	47.6	0.34
1957–1959	3,140	554	143	70.6	29.3	374	49.6	50.4	0.42
1965	3,160	518	145	66.0	34.1	374	48.8	51.2	0.52

From B. Friend, Am. J. Clin. Nutr. 27:1, 1974 and Harold Kahn, Am. J. Clin. Nutr. 23:7, 1970 the same as in 1948, while in 1965, the amount of saturated fat was less than it had been in 1948.

The amount of cholesterol in the daily diet in 1910 was 495 milligrams (561 milligrams in 1948, 554 milligrams in 1958 and in 1965, 518 milligrams). A milligram is one-thousandth of a gram, and since an average egg contains 230 milligrams of cholesterol, the increase in the cholesterol content of the daily diet from 1910 to 1965 was less than the amount contained in one-tenth of an egg. Surely, it seems unlikely that one-seventh of an ounce of saturated fat and one-tenth of an egg added to the 1910 average American daily diet would be sufficient to cause more than 700,000 coronary-thrombosis deaths a year. If one or two eggs a day weren't causing heart attacks in 1900, why should they today?

Be Wary of Those Margarine Ads

Incidentally, the amount of polyunsaturated fats (which occur in margarine, corn oil, soya oil, safflower oil, etc.) nearly doubled from 10.7 grams per day in 1910 (14.8 in 1948 and 16.6 in 1958) to 19.1 in 1965. It would seem that the increase in the polyunsaturated fats in the diet has dismally failed to stop the heart-disease epidemic.

Table 2.5

Yearly per capita consumption of animal fats and vegetable oils.

Year	Butter (lbs.)	Lard (lbs.)	Total Animal Fats (lbs.)	Total Vegetable Oils (lbs.)
1946	10.5	11.8	22.3	14.4
1955	9.0	10.1	19.1	17.7
1963	6.8	6.5	13.3	19.0

U.S.D.A. Report 138 (1969)

In 1971 Americans were dying from coronary thrombosis at a greater rate than the citizens of any other country except Finland. In that year coronary thrombosis killed proportionally five times as many Americans as Japanese; nearly three times as many Americans as Swedes, Swiss, or Italians; and more than twice the number of Dutch, West Germans, or Australians.

In general, the reader should use caution in comparing heart-disease death rate figures from different tables or various researchers, for often the categories included in the survey vary from year to year and from country to country. But Table 2.6, which appeared in *Medical World News,* offers a generally reliable indication of America's unfortunate standing in the heart-disease epidemic in the early 1970s.

Table 2.6

1971 Coronary-Thrombosis Death Rate by Country (per 100,000 population)

Country	Rate
Finland	244.7
U.S.	211.8
Australia	204.6
Canada	187.4
United Kingdom	140.9
The Netherlands	106.9
West Germany	102.3
Austria	88.6
Italy	78.9
Switzerland	75.9
Sweden	74.7
France	41.7
Japan	39.1

Data from *Medical World News,* Feb. 18, 1972

Chances Are You Can Avoid Heart Attack Forever

Because the incidence of heart disease in younger adults varies with lifestyle, it is not inevitable that you get coronary thrombosis, and it is possible to influence your heart health.

Coronary thrombosis, which is now epidemic in the affluent nations, has increased as people have become less active, eaten more proooooood foods, smoked, overeaten, and polluted their environment. It has been reduced recently as people have improved their living habits. But the 10–15 percent reduction in the heart-attack death rate achieved in the last ten years is only a small proportion of the reduction possible.

I believe the principles for heart health explained in later chapters will reduce your odds of developing heart disease before the age of 80 years from 32 percent to less than 3 percent—near the level of that of the generations that ate rich gravies, fatback, whole grains, and fresh vegetables.

Bear in mind what Dr. White emphatically stated (in the 1971 *Family Circle* article previously mentioned): "I believe that *no one* under 70 should be afflicted with heart disease of *any kind.*"

3
The Real Causes
of Heart Disease

Ten to fifteen percent of those with a high risk of developing heart disease avoid the premature death of a coronary. But why is that percentage so low?

Why does heart disease still strike down so many of those that take every precaution advised by the American Heart Association? Consider the case of 47-year-old world-famous heart surgeon Dr. Albert Starr, of the Oregon Medical School in Portland, who needed open-heart surgery and was operated on by the team of physicians he had trained. Dr. Starr, who had performed more than 3,000 such operations himself, had followed all of the well-known guidelines for the prevention of heart disease. He was lean and trim, physically active, a nonsmoker, and his diet conformed to restrictions promoted by the AHA. His diet was low in cholesterol, low in fat, and had the proper ratio of polyunsaturated fats to saturated fats.

Why did 33-year-old, 5'8", 165-pound Harry Moss have a fatal heart attack after jogging only two miles of his regular five-mile jaunt? He was an Alexandria, Virginia, fireman participating in a supervised voluntary physical-fitness program.

Why did two superbly conditioned athletes, former University of Maryland basketball players, die of heart disease in the same year? One, Owen Brown, was 23 years old and the other, Chris Patton, was only 21.

Of course, heredity and congenital defects will explain some of the heart-disease deaths involving those in good physical condition, especially the younger ones. But there are countless cases in which the causes were not primarily hereditary, and where heart disease struck in spite of the fact that all of the AHA recommendations had been followed.

It's Time the AHA Got Off the Anticholesterol Bandwagon

We can reasonably speculate that the AHA has not alerted us to all the heart-disease risk factors. What, in fact, they have not told us is that chemicals added to our food and in our air and water produce dangerous free radicals in the body, which can directly lead to heart disease. Nor have they told us that our diets are deficient in the nutrients (vitamins C and E and the trace mineral selenium) that offer the best protection against the free radicals.

A free radical is a highly reactive molecular fragment. Antioxidants such as vitamin E and the trace mineral selenium deactivate free radicals. Thus the balance between the number of antioxidant molecules and the number of free radicals determines whether the free radicals are controlled (minimized) or not. The greater the balance is upset, either by more sources of free radicals or by fewer antioxidants, the greater the damage. Free radicals generally initiate chain reactions, producing more free radicals and reacted products. One free radical can produce chain reactions altering thousands of molecules.

While the AHA should be alerting us to the full range of risk factors, they should also do whatever they can to halt the cholesterol scare in its tracks. At the moment, there is no indication that they plan to do so.

Chapters 4 through 8 will discuss the recent research that the AHA has ignored—experiments showing that dietary cholesterol is not a major factor in heart disease, and research showing that polyunsaturated fats do not help prevent heart disease.

Chapters 9, 10, and 14 will explain why the antioxidant

vitamins E and C are so important in the prevention of heart disease, although their use has been discounted by the AHA.

Chapter 7 will point out experiments that indicate that avoiding cholesterol and eating a disproportionate amount of polyunsaturated fats is possibly harmful.

It is unfortunate that with good intentions the AHA jumped on the anticholesterol bandwagon too early—before conclusive evidence was obtained—and consequently it is now reluctant to modify its stand, even though modern research dispels the cholesterol myth and reveals the true cause of coronary thrombosis. It's quite likely that they are reluctant to admit they tried the dangerous experiment of changing the nation's diet without conclusive scientific evidence.

The New Theory of Heart Disease

Simply put, coronary thrombosis strikes when two conditions occur at the same time: the first condition is a narrowed artery, the second is sticky blood. The first condition itself can contribute to the second.

The process through which arteries become narrow is called atherosclerosis, and it is a common factor in the various forms of heart disease. "Athera" is the Greek word for "mush," and this is a fair description of the buildup of material called plaque within the arteries. The broadest classification of heart disease is described as "cardiovascular disease" or "coronary heart disease." The more specific problems are described by the following terms:

- *Atherosclerosis*—buildup of plaque in artery walls that narrows the artery.
- *Arteriosclerosis*—hardening of arteries that stiffens them and reduces their flexibility.
- *Ischemia*—reduced blood supply to the heart due to atherosclerosis.
- *Myocardial infarction*—damage to the heart because the

blood supply has been cut off in a region of the heart muscle. This is the epidemic heart attack or coronary (also termed coronary thrombosis because a clot is often found within the heart cavity as well).

- *Angina pectoris*—chest pains produced by ischemia and intensified by physical exertion and stress.
- *Tachycardia*—a regular but very rapid heartbeat, which can be fatal because the heart cannot efficiently deliver blood.
- *Fibrillation*—a weak and chaotic heart action (irregular quiver) which is more serious than tachycardia.
- *Stroke*—blockage of blood to a portion of the brain.
- *Cerebral hemorrhage*—a broken (burst) artery to the brain (often as a result of weakening due to atherosclerosis).
- *Peripheral vascular disease*—the reduction in blood supply to smaller blood vessels, such as those in the extremities.

The narrowed arteries of atherosclerosis are not caused by cholesterol dropping out of the blood onto the artery walls, but by a proliferation of smooth muscle cells in the middle layer of the artery. If the problem were due to high cholesterol levels in the blood, it is likely that several or all of the arteries would have plaques. Instead only one to four arteries are usually involved. In fact, plaques form most frequently near the junction of two arterial branches, as shown in Figures 3.1 through 3.5. If the buildup of plaques were dependent on concentration, it would deposit evenly or on the underside of the junction of the arteries involved. But it doesn't.

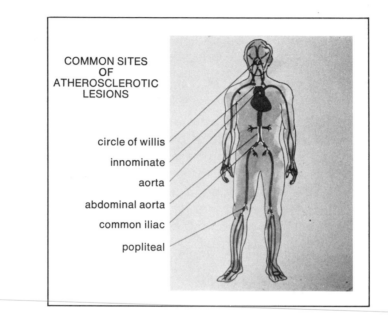

Figure 3.1 COMMON SITES OF ATHEROSCLEROTIC LESIONS
Original drawing by R. Harper. Reprinted with permission of the copyright owner,
Dr. Harold W. Harper.

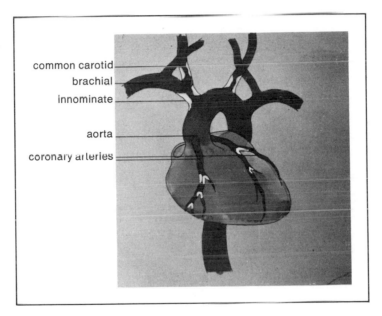

common carotid
brachial
innominate

aorta
coronary arteries

Figure 3.2 Common sites of atherosclerotic lesions: details of coronary sites.
Original drawing by R. Harper. Reprinted with permission of the copyright owner, Dr. Harold W. Harper.

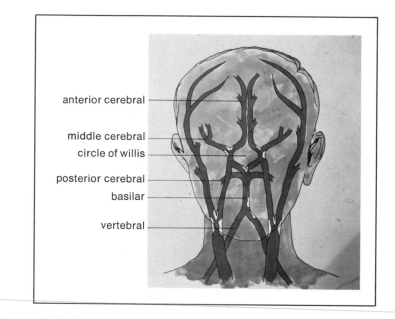

Figure 3.3 Common sites of atherosclerotic lesions: details of head sites.
Original drawing by R. Harper. Reprinted with permission of copyright owner, Dr. Harold W. Harper.

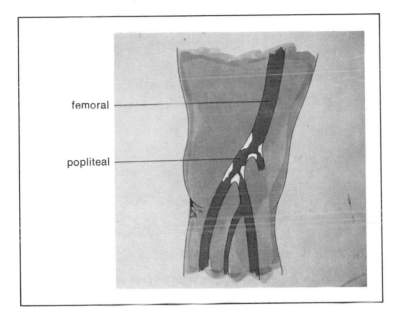

Figure 3.4 Common sites of atherosclerotic lesions: details of leg sites.
Original drawing by R. Harper. Reprinted with permission of copyright owner, Dr. Harold W. Harper.

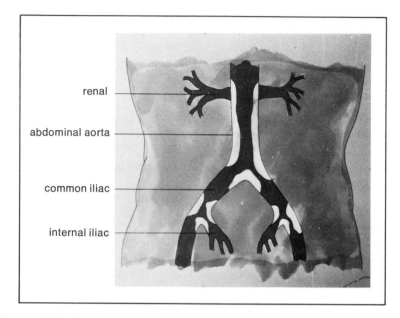

renal

abdominal aorta

common iliac

internal iliac

Figure 3.5 Common sites of atherosclerotic lesions: details of trunk sites.
Original drawing by R. Harper. Reprinted with permission of copyright owner, Dr. Harold W. Harper

The smooth muscle cells of the arteries are stimulated to proliferate (much as in the case where normal cells can become cancer cells and multiply wildly) by chemical mutagens (free radicals, some food additives, some pesticides, and chlorine) and by physical pressure (including high blood pressure) that release potentially harmful chemical factors. Thus the original plaque that builds up in the arteries is fundamentally an accumulation of mutant cells.

In Stage 1 of plaque growth, the proliferating smooth muscle cells spread through the intima (innermost coating of the blood vessel) and is compressed against the endothelium and the internal elastic lamina layers of the artery (see Figure 3.6), causing the production of extracellular substances including collagen (a structural protein) and glycosaminoglycans (a carbohydrate–amino-acid complex).

In Stage 2, these newly formed smooth muscle cells *pro-*

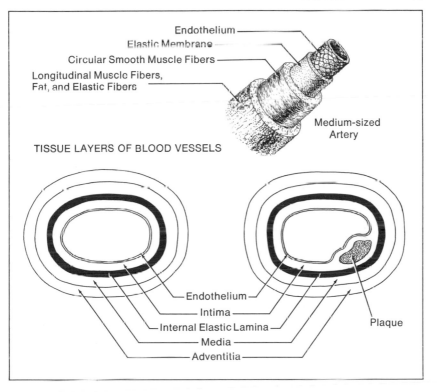

Endothelium

Elastic Membrane

Circular Smooth Muscle Fibers

Longitudinal Muscle Fibers,
Fat, and Elastic Fibers

Medium-sized
Artery

TISSUE LAYERS OF BLOOD VESSELS

Endothelium
Intima
Internal Elastic Lamina
Media
Adventitia

Plaque

Figure 3.6 Common Sites of Atherosclerotic Plaques—The
plaque (or deposit) that forms in the arteries does not form on the
inner surface as is the general belief, but *within* the intima (or
inner layer). In advanced cases of atherosclerosis, the plaque
erupts through the inner surface of the artery and exposes to the
bloodstream the cholesterol and collagen produced by the deterioration of the diseased smooth muscle cells of the artery.

duce and store excessive amounts of cholesterol; and,
eventually, a complicated atherosclerotic plaque is raised in
the artery and erupts through the endothelium into the
lumen.

In Stage 3, electronic charges on the plaque surface at-
tract calcium and cholesterol to the plaque. This process is
independent of blood cholesterol level or dietary cholesterol, for cholesterol would be attracted to the plaque even
if the body's cholesterol supply were so low as to affect the

immediate health of the individual. (Cholesterol is essential to proper functioning of the body; for details see p. 00.)

Each of the steps is controlled by multiple influences including heredity and nutrition. Not surprisingly, a multiple-factor program is required to control this process. The multifactorial program I suggest—The Total Protection Plan—involves six steps. The outline of the plan is presented at the end of the first chapter, and a chart to help you check your progress in following the plan appears in the final chapter.

The evidence implicating the proliferation of smooth muscle cells (technically called the monoclonal origin of atherosclerotic plaques) has been put together by many researchers, but I believe that most of the credit should go to Dr. Earl P. Benditt (Professor and Chairman of the Department of Pathology at the University of Washington School of Medicine at Seattle). Credit is also due Drs. John M. Benditt, N. Moss, J.C.F. Poole, and S.B. Cromwell (all of the University of Washington School of Medicine); Elspeth B. Smith (a University of Aberdeen pathologist); and Robert H. Heptinstall (of the Johns Hopkins University School of Medicine). For those interested in following this radical new explanation for atherosclerosis—first proposed in 1970 but unconfirmed until 1975—the eleven articles listed in Appendix 10 will be helpful.

The implications of this new explanation are far-reaching. First they show that cholesterol has little to do with plaque formation, and second they show that the origins of heart disease share certain similarities with the origins of cancer. That is, harmful substances in our air, water, and food, and a decrease in the nutritive value of our diets, cause the cellular damage that prepares the way for both diseases. Dr. Robert I. Levy, director of the National Heart, Lung, and Blood Institute, offered the following remarks to me in a 1976 letter. He presents a balanced overlook of the monoclonal-proliferation theory, and his entire letter is reproduced in Appendix 1.

"Certainly the Benditt study has been a most imaginative and stimulating one. The basic observation that the raised fibrous or fibro-fatty plaques are predominantly monoclonal appears to be firmly established by the work of Benditt and his colleagues, by work from Heptinstall's laboratory at Johns Hopkins, and by the work from Thomas's laboratory at Albany. . . . It is probably fair to say that additional data will need to be obtained before the question can be resolved to everyone's satisfaction."

The Experiments That Led to the Discovery

Let's look at Dr. Earl Benditt's discovery that a group of identical cells originating from a single cell produces the atherosclerotic plaque. In 1970, Benditt and his colleagues reported that atherosclerotic plaques formed spontaneously in chickens, and closely resembled those in humans. This, in itself, was an important discovery, because plaques can be caused in experimental animals, such as rabbits, by feeding them extremely high amounts of cholesterol; but the plaques so formed do not resemble the plaques found in people with heart disease. Similarly, plaquelike material can form in experimental animals when an artery is irritated or injured purposely by a surgical device called a balloon catheter, yet these plaquelike formations also do not resemble the atherosclerotic plaques in humans. The most important finding, however, was that the plaques found in some chickens consisted of a small population of cells which differed from the cells in healthy chicken arteries or in arteries experimentally injured.

Next, Dr. Benditt and his colleagues examined cells in human plaques and in healthy human arteries in a sophisticated manner. They found that the cells in human atherosclerotic plaques were different from the cells in healthy human arteries, just as they had found in their examination of chickens.

It is important to note that evidence supporting the monoclonal-proliferation explanation of heart disease comes from studies of human plaques. Proponents of other explanations of heart disease do not have direct evidence from human studies, but rather inferences from animal studies.

In 1973, Dr. Benditt and co-workers discovered that the individual cells of the atherosclerotic plaques in humans were all identical, although normal cells are not. This observation suggested a common genetic origin for the plaque cells. Additionally, they found in healthy arteries two forms of the enzyme G-6-PD (glucose-6-phosphate dehydrogenase), although in the plaques only one or the other form appeared—never both.

They further found that the proliferating cells are smaller and produce primarily collagen, whereas normal artery cells produce primarily elastin. And they found that the proliferating cells also differ in the composition of the extracellular material produced by their injury-repair cells. Lastly they found that the proliferating cells are not as well arranged as normal cells. These observations were confirmed by Dr. Heptinstall's group. (See Appendix 10.) The findings suggested that the single cell from which the plaque cells had proliferated had become genetically transformed (as a result of mutation) from normal artery cells.

The cholesterol found in the cells of the deeper layers of the plaque and in the atheromatous debris underlying the plaques is probably produced by the cells in response to cellular injury. The cells in the deepest layers frequently appear to be dying and disintegrating. This finding was also confirmed by Dr. Heptinstall's group.

You may ask why all previous researchers had missed these observations. Perhaps it was because newly developed, sophisticated techniques and a great deal of detective work were required for their discovery. Or perhaps others saw only the cholesterol and assumed that the monoclonal cells were just part of the material eroded from the artery along with the cholesterol. When you set out to prove that cholesterol is the villain, you can overlook a lot of facts inconsistent with the anticholesterol myth.

The Final Step in Plaque Formation—Calcification

An equally important consideration is that once cholesterol has been produced within the fibrous plaque, the cholesterol attracts calcium from the blood stream. The calcium is held to the plaque by electrical-charge attraction, and the addition of the calcium hardens the plaque, much as rivets or nails add rigidity to structures.

The plaque-building process continues as the calcium attracts additional material from the bloodstream, including cholesterol, triglycerides, and carotene. This attraction is again a charge-gradient attraction (this time coming from the powerful intrinsic charge of positive divalent calcium). Although the cholesterol and lipids (fatty materials) are electrically neutral, they have regions of polarity, much like a magnet. Thus, with positive attracting negative, and negative attracting positive, the plaque will grow in size as layer after layer is added.

It is important to realize that the cholesterol attracted by the calcium will come from the bloodstream, even when cholesterol levels are low. It is not a concentration-controlled process, but a charge-controlled process.

Some investigators ignore the charge-controlled aspect and concentrate on lipoprotein fractions in the bloodstream. (Lipoproteins are a group of eight different substances that carry cholesterol through the bloodstream.) These investigators are more interested in the amount of cholesterol which blood can make soluble in addition to the cholesterol already present. This ability is called the serum cholesterol binding reserve (SCBR), and it is determined by its lipoprotein subfractions.

Dr. William P. Castelli, Director of Laboratories for the Framingham group, points out that the ratio of two particular lipoprotein fractions is the most important factor in protection against heart disease. The high density lipoprotein (HDL), carries cholesterol (sometimes called alpha-cholesterol fraction) from the tissues to the liver for excretion. Eskimos have high HDL levels but rarely suffer from heart disease because of HDL's protective effect.

Dr. Castelli remarked during a 1977 Science Writer's Seminar, "I've seen a woman who was being treated for high cholesterol, but when we tested her, we found that she had lots of HDL, but very little LDL. (LDL, Low Density Lipoprotein, is another lipoprotein fraction having the opposite effect of unloading cholesterol into the tissues.) That patient will outlive her doctor—and all of us."

Out of 2,400 men and women free of heart disease at the start of Dr. Castelli's study eight years ago, 79 new cases of heart disease developed among the men. All but nine of these men had low HDL levels.

In Dr. Castelli's study men with HDL levels of 25 mg% (milligrams per deciliter of blood) or less had a heart attack rate of 176.5 per 1,000, while those with levels between 65–74 mg%, had a ratio of only 25 heart attacks per 1,000. *However, men in Dr. Castelli's study with HDL levels above 75 mg% had no heart attacks at all.*

Reviewing the processes involved shows that there are three major stages of the primary plaque development that produce clinical symptoms of cardiovascular disease. Stage 1 involves monoclonal proliferation, stage 2 the formation of cholesterol within the fibrous plaque, and stage 3 the formation of hardened layers of calcium and cholesterol via electrical-charge attraction. Appendix 2 discusses how the injury-caused plaques as well as harmless, non-symptomatic plaques are formed by other processes. Such plaques are relatively unimportant.

Evidence will be presented in subsequent chapters to show that stage 1 can be prevented by antioxidant nutrients, and that stage 3 can be reversed naturally by low-calorie diets, the Dr. Rinse Breakfast, and vitamin C. More rapid reversal, which may be necessary in advanced stages of atherosclerosis, can be accomplished by chelation therapy. (See Chapter 30.)

High Blood Pressure and Cigarette Smoke Can Start the Cholesterol-Producing Process

Other heart-disease risk factors, in addition to environmental chemicals, are involved in promoting the cell proliferation. High blood pressure causes physical injury to arterial cells which, in turn, release certain chemicals into the artery to start the healing process. These chemicals can cause the cell proliferation, and are often mutagenic (causing a slightly different cell to be produced).

Cigarette smoke in the bloodstream can also initiate cell proliferation, by causing aryl hydrocarbons (including the mutagen and carcinogen benzopyrene) to be released into the bloodstream. (An interesting fact is that an enzyme involved in the cigarette-smoke mutagen/carcinogen process is preferentially carried in the same vehicle [lipoprotein] in the blood as cholesterol. This could account for the minor association of heart disease with a high blood cholesterol level. A person can genetically have a high level of the vehicle that carries both the cholesterol and the enzyme [AHH] that causes the cell proliferation. Thus some investigators might falsely associate the plaque formation with cholesterol level in the blood, rather than with the mutagen/carcinogen level.)

Factors released from blood platelets (see Chapter 9) can also cause the mutation. Vitamin E can reduce the release of these blood-platelet factors, thus lowering the risk of heart disease. Exercise and diet can control the health of the arteries, as well as positively influence the intrinsic chemicals that can cause proliferation.

A possible link between low-level radiation (a source of free radicals) and heart disease has been suggested by Dr. K.T. Lee of the Albany, New York, Medical College. Pigs given a high-fat diet plus doses of radiation rapidly develop atherosclerosis and die. Pigs on the same diet but without the radiation do not develop the atherosclerosis.

The Real Risk Factors

Medical researchers have blamed the heart-disease epidemic on a variety of factors. Included in their lists have been:

1) excessive intake of cholesterol,
2) excessive intake of saturated fats,
3) cigarette smoking,
4) Type A personality or stress,
5) lack of exercise,
6) lack of roughage (fiber),
7) excessive calories,
8) diabetes,
9) hypothyroidism,
10) heredity,
11) age,
12) sex,
13) high blood triglycerides,
14) high blood beta-lipoproteins,
15) chlorine in the drinking water,
16) soft water,
17) excessive sugar,
18) coffee,
19) alcohol,
20) vitamin deficiencies,
21) mineral deficiencies,
22) meat,
23) an enzyme in homogenized cow's milk,
24) environmental pollutants, and
25) high blood pressure.

The list of risk factors proposed by the National Heart, Lung, and Blood Institute is short—in fact, not inclusive enough. That institute reports that their physicians are not yet sure which risk factors are the most dangerous, but they do agree on one point: the more factors present in a person, the greater the risk of a heart attack or stroke. (See figure 3.7.) Their list is as follows:

1) too much of fatty substances—particularly cholesterol or triglycerides—in the blood,
2) high blood pressure,
3) cigarette smoking,
4) diabetes,
5) obesity,
6) rapid or markedly irregular pulse,
7) sedentary living with little exercise,
8) family history of heart attacks or strokes, and
9) emotional tension

The American Heart Association lists similar risks and recommends cutting cholesterol and saturated fats, and increasing the ratio of polyunsaturated fats to saturated fats.

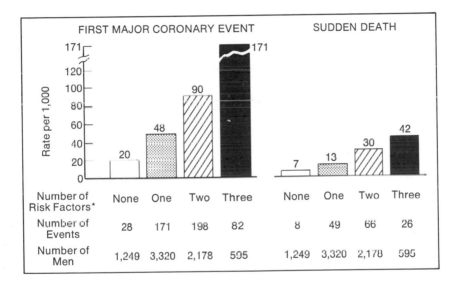

Figure 3.7 The more risk factors that are present in a person, the greater the risk of heart attack or stroke. From Stamler and Epstein (*Preventive Medicine,* 1972).

In the United Kingdom, the Advisory Panel of the Committee on Medical Aspects of Food Policy (Nutrition) on Diet in

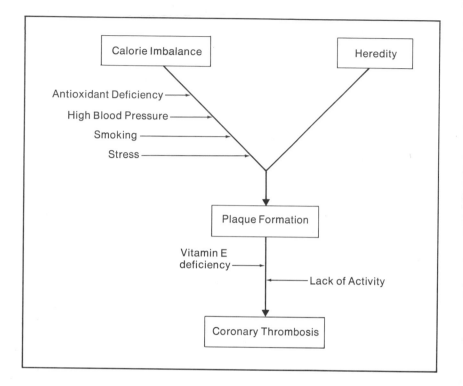

Figure 3.8 Major pathway to coronary thrombosis. The path to a heart attack is a two-step process. First a plaque is formed in the artery interior and then a clot is formed at the plaque site when the blood becomes sticky. Note that dietary cholesterol is not a factor. Calorie imbalance means you eat too much for your level of activity; it does not indicate a lack of exercise.

Relation to Cardiovascular and Cerebrovascular Disease recommends the following to diminish the risk of heart disease (although the importance of each factor is not known):

1) obesity should be avoided
2) the amount of fats consumed should be reduced. (The panel unanimously agreed that they could not recommend an increase in the intake of polyunsaturated fats.)
3) the amount of sugar should be reduced

4) proposals for softening the community water supply should be opposed.

Figure 3.8 shows what I believe are the seven real risk factors and how they are involved in the development of heart disease.

In order for a "potential risk factor" to qualify as a "real risk factor," it must increase the incidence of heart disease above that of a second risk factor, when both risk factors are combined. As an example, dietary cholesterol fails to affect the heart-disease rate when added to smoking or high blood pressure, or any other factor; thus it doesn't qualify as a real risk factor.

Heredity is, however, a major risk factor, but one that cannot be controlled. What we can do is try to control the other six factors.

4
Behind the Cholesterol Myth

Avoiding cholesterol is the worst form of food-faddism, yet it has received the blessing of the American Heart Association. As a result of continuous advertising to that effect, Americans have been conditioned to avoid cholesterol-containing foods, although avoiding cholesterol may do more harm than good.

Crude, oversimplified, and inaccurate studies from the 1940s and 1950s are largely responsible for the popular concept that a high consumption of saturated fats may cause elevated levels of cholesterol in the blood or increased risk of heart disease. But many more recent studies conducted under better-controlled conditions (and with more accurate analysis of blood levels of cholesterol) show either no correlation at all, or a weak correlation. A number of these studies show that there is less heart disease and longer life among those eating normal amounts of cholesterol and fats. Furthermore, several studies indicated that those on some low-cholesterol diets developed more serious illnesses, including cancer and heart disease itself.

The task of reeducation is difficult. As Dr. Michael Oliver (of the Department of Cardiology of the Royal Infirmary in Edinburgh) puts it: "Many who study cardiovascular epidemiology, nutrition, or cardiology have neither the will, the wish, nor the time to examine the fabric of the case for or against causal relationships. Opinions are set and deaf ears are turned. The polarization of views in the United States, for example, goes so far as to result in major court actions, alienation between doctors, disagreements within families, excessive advertising, and missionary zeal. Sometimes the advocates of a significant relation between, for example, dietary fat and coronary heart disease speak so loudly and so often that they endanger their own good case by appearing to be uncritical and to overlook inconvenient facts." (*British Heart Journal,* 1976.)

Dr. Oliver further points out in the same article that "the evidence incriminating dietary cholesterol as a cause of coronary heart disease in developed countries is virtually non-existent."

Scientists can now draw only one conclusion. "The inescapable conclusion is that the lipid (fat and cholesterol) hypothesis is based on unsound evidence.... The lipid hypothesis and the evidence on which it is based are so rife with variable results and inconsistencies that there is need for the protagonists of the lipid theory to review the premises on which their beliefs depend and for strict adherence to concrete, indisputable facts." (Stehbens, *Cardiovascular Medicine,* March 1977.)

Another researcher puts it more strongly. "The hypothesis that saturated fats and cholesterol cause coronary heart disease—a proposal raised before 1950 on shaky evidence —has been repeatedly tested and *found wrong."* (Dr. George V. Mann in *Meat and Health Series No. 2,* National Live Stock and Meat Board, 1976.)

Even practicing physicians, who have long been dismayed as their patients on strict low-cholesterol diets continue to suffer heart attacks, are speaking out. One example is a Lancaster, Pennsylvania, physician: "As stated by Corday and Corday in their recent review of the subject, the time has come to face the facts. The lipid hypothesis—that lipids cause arterial disease and that lowering lipids will decrease arterial disease—is no longer viable and should be recognized as such. I am not disparaging the great amount of work done on the problem but, rather, saying it is time to accept that the problem has not been substantiated." (Dr. H. Newland, *Annals of Internal Medicine,* 1976.)

The Origin of the Cholesterol Myth

The cholesterol myth started in 1862 when Virchow postulated fat infiltration as the cause of arterial deposits. In 1913 a Russian scientist, Dr. Nikolai Anitschkov, found that feeding high amounts of crystalline cholesterol to rabbits could induce heart disease in the rabbits. What he failed to realize was that rabbits are vegetarians and their systems cannot handle cholesterol-containing animal foods, let alone crystalline cholesterol. He also failed to realize that the deposits formed by feeding rabbits cholesterol are different from the plaques formed in man. The deposits in rabbit arteries are free of the fibrous material found in human plaques. And, as explained in Appendix 2, it's only fibrous plaques that contribute to heart disease.

Since then, hundreds of millions of dollars have been spent attempting to prove that dietary cholesterol can induce heart disease in man. Many of these research funds have come from commercial interests which manufacture cereals and polyunsaturated-fat products. And many millions more will continue to be spent to reinforce the erroneous claim.

Cholesterol Performs Important Functions

Much of the early speculation about cholesterol was done by physicians who lacked in-depth biochemical training. Consequently, they did not realize that you don't have to eat cholesterol for cholesterol to be present in the body. The body can produce cholesterol from protein, carbohydrates, or fats. And this is fortunate, for cholesterol is necessary in several internal processes. The presence of cholesterol is essential in order for your nerves to transmit their impulses throughout your body. Cholesterol is converted into various hormones, including the sex hormones. It is also made into bile, is incorporated into cellular membranes, and has an important function in the brain. The blood vessels themselves make cholesterol to provide lubrication.

If you were to completely avoid eating cholesterol, your body would still produce as much as you needed, even if you were fasting. In fact, your body will manufacture cholesterol at the expense of many other constituents if there is a shortage. Because a feedback mechanism senses your need for cholesterol and the amount available, your body will make less cholesterol when you eat more.

Cholesterol Levels in the Blood Are Regulated Naturally

As long ago as 1953, it was known that you couldn't overload the bloodstream with cholesterol for more than a short time after consuming large quantities of cholesterol. A report in the *Journal of Mt. Sinai Hospital* (N.Y.) in that year showed that blood cholesterol will rise after a person eats a large quantity of cholesterol, but within a few hours will return to the level maintained before eating. It is important to remember that, when your blood cholesterol is measured in a routine physical examination, the blood sample is taken after a fast of 10 to 12 hours. Therefore, if the reading is high, it is not due to the temporary effect of eating.

In the Mt. Sinai experiment, *ten grams* of cholesterol (equivalent to the amount in 45 eggs) were given to 73 healthy men along with a breakfast of scrambled eggs, butter, toast, coffee, and cream. Blood cholesterol levels in the men being tested rose to a peak within four hours following administration of this massive dose, and returned to normal within 24 hours. You would think that if 3 eggs a week were the reasonable limit (as the American Heart Association keeps telling us), the cholesterol equivalent of 45 eggs in one meal would have caused cholesterol to settle out of the blood and fill the arteries in the legs up past knee level, like mud settling from dirty water.

As the Mt. Sinai study indicates, fear about cholesterol buildup in the body as a result of eating cholesterol-rich foods is groundless. Yet cholesterolphobia is depriving many Americans of good nutrition. Most low-cholesterol

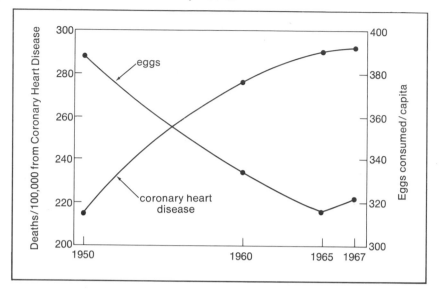

Figure 4.1 Correlation between egg consumption and deaths from heart disease.

Based on a Paper presented at the Eighth Annual Colorado Poultry Institute Meeting, March 1971, by Dr. Byron F. Miller entitled *Cholesterol kickback.* (Also see R. H. Hall, *Food for Nought,* Harper and Row, New York, 1974)

diets are not properly balanced (especially in regard to selenium, lecithin, iron, phosphorus, vitamins A and B₂, and, less frequently, essential amino acids). This undernutrition is a cause of heart disease, cancer, and other serious health problems.

Cholesterol-Theory Flaws

The theory that a high-cholesterol diet causes heart disease has always had serious flaws. If the theory were valid, why are there cities in the U.S. having twice the heart-disease death rate of other cities nearly equally matched in activity and diet? One explanation is that the incidence of heart disease correlates more with the hardness or softness of the drinking water than with diet. (See Chapter 16.)

And why, if high cholesterol causes heart disease, do people not exhibiting the classical risk factors develop heart disease? Studies by Drs. Ray H. Rosenman and Meyer Friedman (authors of *Type A Behavior and Your Heart,* Knopf, 1974) have shown that a substantial number of men who developed heart disease were free of all of the popular risk factors.

Drs. Rosenman and Friedman have further observed that blood cholesterol levels in most of their heart patients are lower than the normal limit. The upper limit of normal is considered to be 300 mg/100 ml, yet they found that 62 percent of their patients had cholesterol levels below 260 mg/100 ml. Additionally, they found that both cholesterol and blood pressure were normal in half of their heart patients, while both factors were abnormal in only one in ten of their heart patients.

In summary they said, "Evaluation of these data led us to conclude that neither diet, serum lipids (including cholesterol and triglycerides), nor any other recognized risk factor was essentially responsible for the increase in coronary morbidity observed during the past few decades in industrialized societies." These findings led them to their study of stress and personality types. (See Chapter 29.)

Dr. Michael DeBakey, one of America's foremost heart surgeons, and his research group found similar results. Here is a significant passage from their report: "An analysis of cholesterol values by usual hospital laboratory methods in 1,700 patients with atherosclerotic disease revealed no definite correlation between serum cholesterol levels and the nature and extent of atherosclerotic disease. Eight out of ten [heart] patients had cholesterol values below the upper limits of normal for the procedure employed." (H.E. Garrett, E. C. Horning, B. G. Creech, and M. DeBakey, *Journal of the American Medical Association,* 1964.) In 1976 the analysis was updated with results again showing no definite correlation.

Many other questions haunt the cholesterol theory:

- Why do low-cholesterol diets designed to prevent heart disease in experimental animals actually cause heart disease?
- Why do seals and walruses, who eat primarily an unsaturated-fat diet, develop arterial plaques nearly identical to man's?
- Why are fibrous plaques found only in arteries, whereas cholesterol levels are the same in veins and arteries? When veins are surgically transplanted to serve as arteries, they too develop plaque—even on low-cholesterol diets. Since clots form in both veins and arteries, why are the plaques irregularly distributed? If blood cholesterol levels are the same throughout the body, the deposits would be expected to be generally distributed.
- Hemodynamic (or blood hydrodynamic) laws explain the site probabilities which correspondingly fit very well into the monoclonal-proliferation explanation of heart disease. (See Figures 3.1 through 3.5 and Appendix 1.)
- Why, although the blood cholesterol level suddenly increases only slightly in women following menopause, does the heart-disease incidence in women past menopause increase 300 percent?
- Why is heart disease in swine characterized by fibrous plaque without a trace of cholesterol, unless artifically caused extremely high blood cholesterol levels from an abnormal diet saturate the plaque?

There are many more "holes" in the cholesterol theory, but let's look directly at the studies that falsely pinpointed cholesterol in the first place, and at the studies that now prove the cholesterol theory to be false.

Framingham Conclusion Proves Cholesterol Is Not a Cause of Heart Disease

But the Framingham Study is the study that everyone uses to prove we shouldn't eat cholesterol, isn't it?

That's right. The American Heart Association relies heavily on "evidence" from the Framingham Study. But, despite the study's multitude of flaws, its conclusion did prove that dietary cholesterol does not cause heart disease; in fact, it showed that, if anything, people eating normal amounts of cholesterol have lower heart-disease risk.

The report released in 1970 at the termination of the Framingham Study shocked most heart researchers that read it. Unfortunately, most physicians didn't read it, as they assumed it was just one more Framingham report warning of the alleged dangers of cholesterol.

The report (made by Dr. William B. Kannel, Director of the project, and Tavia Gordon, a National Heart, Lung, and Blood Institute statistician), studied 437 men and 475 women for periods up to ten years, and concluded that no matter how much or how little animal fat there is in the diet, some people will have low levels of cholesterol in their blood, others will have moderate levels, and still others high levels. The report specifically emphasized that there was "no suggestion of any relation between diet and the subsequent development of coronary heart disease in the study group, despite a distinct elevation of serum cholesterol in men developing coronary heart disease."

The Flaws in the Framingham Study

The Framingham Study, begun in 1948, was an imperfect design, carried out in a questionable fashion, and misinterpreted by those with preconceived notions that dietary cholesterol was the cause of heart disease.

It is surprising that so many researchers and physicians accepted the early Framingham conclusions implicating cholesterol as a cause of heart disease, despite the absence of any straight-line relation between the blood cholesterol level and heart-disease death rate.

Most people think that the anxious monitoring of cholesterol levels is a recent practice of modern medicine, but it is really a holdover from the popular medicine of the 1940s and 1950s. Unfortunately, reliability is only now coming to cholesterol measurements. As Dr. Ed Pinckney shows in his book *The Cholesterol Controversy,* improperly applying a tourniquet raises the cholesterol level. Still, relying on cholesterol levels to indicate heart-disease risk is outdated, and so are the early Framingham reports. They should be buried, and only the last report by Kannel and Gordon saved for posterity.

Three of the best critiques of the Framingham reports were done by Dr. Lars Werko, a World Health Organization scientist from Göteborg, Sweden (in *American Heart Journal,* 1976); Dr. Kurt Oster, Chief of Cardiology, Park City Hospital, Bridgeport, Connecticut (in *Medical Counterpoint,* 1972); and Stephen A. Bauman, a consulting mathematician (in *Medical Counterpoint,* 1972).

Dr. Werko questioned the inclusion in the group studied of those with questionable symptoms or signs of disease which were not defined, and the lack of control of patient treatment. Although no treatment was administrated through the study group, the participants' personal physicians were notified of the findings in the first investigation and were free to administer any type of treatment they saw fit. If, how, or to what extent such treatment influenced the results was unclear.

In all, 2,283 men were selected for the study. Dr. Werko observed that "Early in the study, it was clear that the sample could not be considered to represent the American male population. . . . The distribution of blood pressure and serum cholesterol in the population studied in Framingham differs from what has been reported for United States white males. It must also be obvious that the participating families in Framingham do not reflect the wide socioeconomic range of the American community. . . . It was found that the mortality from coronary heart disease in the Framingham sample was different from the mortality in the community."

Dr. Werko also criticized the inclusion of volunteer participants with those selected at random. British experience in multiphasic health screening has indicated a difference in sickness and mortality between volunteer participants and random selections, and that experience proved out in the Framingham Study. There was a rather marked difference in cardiovascular and total mortality rates between the volunteers and selectees.

"These considerations regarding the mode of selection of the populations for the Framingham Study," Dr. Werko commented, "thus lead to the conclusion that any result of this study is only applicable to that part of the population of the city of Framingham that has taken part in the study. . . . Instead, research workers of all kinds have used the Framingham data as if it represented the male population not only in the USA, but in the whole Western Industrialized part of the world."

Dr. Kurt Oster also questioned the study. He was notably unimpressed with the accuracy and reliability of the cholesterol measurements. Cholesterol measurements should be taken after eight to ten hours of fasting, but this wasn't always (if ever) done in the study. "The Framingham blood specimens were taken when convenient to the volunteers regardless of diet, time of day, or other anamnestic influences. . . ."

Dr. Oster's most serious objections, however, deal with the erroneous, unfounded mathematical formula applied to the cholesterol data (already of doubtful value) to correlate with the incidence of heart disease. Stephen Bauman added more criticisms to the misapplication of statistical treatments.

I realize that it is considered virtually sacrilegious to attack the Framingham Study, but when nearly 1 million Americans die each year from heart disease and stroke, it's time to set the facts straight.

The National Pooling Project

Another study sometimes quoted in support of the cholesterol myth is the National Pooling Project. It raises even more questions.

In an attempt to get data from larger populations, several U.S. studies pooled their data in 1970, but the various differences in techniques and definitions caused many problems. Oddly, the number of participants varies from 7,342 to 7,594 in different tables. In one instance a comparison of Table A and Table B indicated a difference of 110 heart attacks among 85 men. This sort of discrepancy makes one uneasy about the quality of the project.

The most important observation that can be made from a study of the Pooling Project is that the addition of high blood cholesterol levels to only one of the other risk factors does not seem to increase the risk of heart disease.

Dr. Werko said of the National Pooling Project, "Regardless of the lack of proof that it is the American diet that causes an elevation of serum cholesterol in the population samples studied, the discussion focuses on the necessity of changing the diet of the general population. . . . It seems, then, rather remarkable that the involved authors—and official bodies—continue to stress high serum cholesterol and diet as *the* risk factor that has to be controlled through general and individual intervention."

Ten years before conclusions of the Pooling Project were published, a report in the Canadian Medical Association's *Journal* found no relationship between blood cholesterol and atherosclerosis. But, of course, it was ignored.

5

Dietary Cholesterol
Is Not the Problem

In the 1960s, while the American Heart Association was calling for the reduction of fats and cholesterol in the diets of all Americans, the American Medical Association (AMA) was still unconvinced. A press release issued by the AMA in 1962 offered the following warning: "The anti-fat, anti-cholesterol fad is not just foolish and futile . . . it also carries some risk.

"Scientific reports linking cholesterol and heart attacks have touched off a new food fad among do-it-yourself Americans. But dieters who believe they can cut down on their blood cholesterol without medical supervision are in for a rude awakening. It could even be dangerous to try."

The AMA's Council on Foods and Nutrition made this observation in 1965: "It must be recalled that definitive proof that lowering serum cholesterol, or preventing a rise in serum cholesterol, will lower the morbidity [illness] and mortality associated with coronary heart disease, is still lacking."

It seems that not everyone was misled by the early Framingham reports, but those who "intuitively" felt the reports were right or who had financial gains at stake broadcast the erroneous conclusions loudly and widely.

For example, in a public statement in 1958 the American Society for the Study of Arteriosclerosis announced, "High blood cholesterol was a definite cause of coronary-artery disease." Doctors, as well as health organizations, were sounding the alarm. In one of many such remarks, Dr.

Thomas R. Dawber reiterated, "There is convincing evidence that [blood] cholesterol levels are definitely related, both to the presence . . . and the development . . . of coronary heart disease." (*Modern Concepts of Cardiovascular Disease,* 1961.)

To date, the most effective voice of opposition has been the book *The Cholesterol Controversy* by Edward R. Pinckney, M.D., and Cathey Pinckney (Sherbourne Press, 1973). Dr. Pinckney first wrote about the lack of specificity of cholesterol in 1957 as an editorial in the *Journal of the American Medical Association.* I first spoke out on the issue in *American Laboratory* in 1972. But, despite criticism, for years the Framingham study has inspired the zealots and opportunists who wanted the nutritious staples eggs, milk, butter, and meats removed from our diets.

Eating Eggs Does Not Cause High Cholesterol

Although early Framingham reports suggested only questionable association between cholesterol consumption and heart disease, wide pronouncements were soon made by numerous doctors, researchers, and the AHA to avoid eggs. Yet no tests on eggs had been conducted. It takes only a month or two to determine whether eating eggs affects cholesterol levels in the blood, but the Framingham researchers and others had no plans whatsoever to test this premise before preaching about their intuitive conclusion. Apparently it didn't occur to them that their ancestors had eaten eggs for thousands of years without developing coronary thrombosis!

In 1975, a research team headed by Dr. Roslyn Alfin-Slater (of the University of California at Los Angeles) set about to perform just such tests. The researchers selected two groups of healthy male subjects who normally ate eggs and whose serum cholesterol and blood pressure were in the normal range. One group, 25 men whose age ranged from 20 to 28 years, were fed two eggs per day for eight weeks *in addition* to their usual cholesterol-containing diet.

The other group, 27 men with an age range of 39 to 66 years, were fed one egg a day for four weeks, then two eggs every other day for four weeks, in addition to their usual cholesterol-containing diet. For two weeks after the eight-week feeding period, all eggs were removed from the diets of both groups.

Serum cholesterol determinations were conducted in each of two successive weeks before the egg diets were begun, weekly for eight weeks during the egg feeding, and thereafter once each week during the two weeks of the egg-free diet. The results indicate that there were no significant differences in average serum cholesterol levels between any two time periods in either group. This research, reported at the International Congress of Nutrition in Kyoto, Japan, in 1975, surprised even the UCLA researchers themselves.

A *Los Angeles Times* article on October 2, 1975, quoted Dr. Alfin-Slater: "We, like everyone else, had been convinced that when you eat cholesterol, you get cholesterol. But when we stopped to think that all of the studies in the past never tested the normal diet in relation to egg eating, and that most were highly controlled in protein, fat, and cholesterol regulation, we decided to see what happened to cholesterol levels of normal diets when egg intake was increased. Our finding [of no increase in blood cholesterol] surprised us as much as ever."

Dr. Alfin-Slater continued, "We hope the study makes people less afraid of eggs. We know the American Heart Association is sincere in its effort to offset the risk of heart disease by recommending restrictions in cholesterol consumption. But eggs are not poison. They are a good food."

The UCLA results were confirmed in 1976 by Professor A. H. Ismail of Purdue University, who tested a group of 24 healthy men between the ages of 21 and 67. Each man ate one additional egg a day compared to his original diet. Dr. Ismail found no effect on blood cholesterol levels in the men. No rise in blood cholesterol levels were found in patients with severe burns receiving 35 eggs each day for up to two months. Burn patients need more calories because large areas of skin are gone and the body loses heat. They also need large amounts of protein to build new skin. The researchers thought that they might be raising the patients' cholesterol levels, but were surprised to learn that the cholesterol levels were normal (Dr. B. Hirshowitz et al., *British Journal of Plastic Surgery,* 1976).

Dr. Peter N. Herbert, chief of clinical service in the Molecular Disease Branch of the National Heart, Lung, and Blood Institute, said his study of patients with normal and elevated cholesterol levels showed that the yolks of six to eight eggs (40 grams) added daily to a therapeutic diet produced no significant rise in blood cholesterol. The results of this study appear unequivocal (*Medical World News,* February 1977).

In England, the Report of the Advisory Panel of the Committee on Medical Aspects of Food Policy on Diet in Relation to Cardiovascular and Cerebrovascular Disease observed, "Most of the dietary cholesterol in western communities is derived from eggs, but we have found no evidence which relates the number of eggs consumed to a risk of coronary heart disease." Furthermore, they state, "The Panel unanimously agree that they cannot recommend an increase in the intake of polyunsaturated fatty acids in the diet as a measure intended to reduce the risk of the development of ischemic [coronary] heart disease. In their opinion the available evidence that such a dietary alteration would reduce the risk in the United Kingdom at the present time is not convincing. In the present state of knowledge any suggestion or claim to that effect, with respect to the nation or to an individual, would be unjustified." (*Diet and Coronary Heart Disease,* London, 1974.)

Significantly, the World Health Organization reported after a 15-year period ending in 1973 that heart-disease deaths in Japan decreased 14 percent while egg consumption went up 300 percent. In the same period the American heart-disease death rate went up 20 percent while our egg consumption went down 20 percent.

In August of 1976 at a special workshop at the Fourth International Symposium on Atherosclerosis (in Japan), the body of scientists from around the world concluded that there should be no restriction on egg intake in a population group with normal cholesterol metabolism.

Dietary Fat Doesn't Raise Cholesterol Either!

Well, if eggs don't cause high serum cholesterol, how about fat? The answer is there's no relationship in normal people unless they're eating too many calories.

In Tecumseh, Michigan, a study of dietary habits revealed that there was no relationship between eating cholesterol, saturated fats, or any of 110 different food items. In this study of 4,057 adults representing more than 90 percent of the adult population of Tecumseh, the researchers found that the only positive correlation with heart disease was excess body fat. Blood cholesterol and triglyceride values did not correlate with dietary constituents. However, a statistically significant relationship was found between the blood cholesterol and triglyceride levels and adiposity (excessive body fat).

The researchers concluded, "These findings suggest that blood cholesterol and triglyceride levels among Americans are more dependent on degree of adiposity than on frequency of consumption of fat, sugar, starch, or alcohol. ... From the findings in this study, one may infer that weight reduction should be the initial intervention for control of hyperlipidemia [elevated blood fats] in the general population." Again we note calorie balance as the most important factor. This important study was conducted by Drs. A. B. Nichols, C. Ravenscroft, D. E. Lamphiear, and L. D. Ostrander, and published in the October 26, 1976 issue of the *Journal of the American Medical Association*.

Several studies of populations having little or no heart disease have been conducted, and it has been discovered that some of the groups eat food very high in saturated fats and cholesterol. Such groups include:

- the Maasai of Tanzania (G. V. Mann et al., *Journal of Atherosclerosis Research*, 1964),

- the Samburu and Punjabis of Northern Kenya (A. G. Shaper, *American Heart Journal,* 1962),
- the Swiss of the Loetschental Valley (Gsell, Detal, *American Journal of Clinical Nutrition,* 1962),
- the Benedictine monks (G. V. Mann, *Nutrition Reviews,* 1963),
- the Northern Indians (S. L. Malhotra, *American Journal of Atherosclerosis Research,* 1964),
- the primitive Eskimos (Vilhjalmur Stefansson in *Cancer: Disease of Civilization,* Greenwood, Ill., 1943),
- the Atiu and Mitiaro natives of Polynesia, (J. D. Hunter, *Federation Proceedings* 21:36, 1962),
- the Jews living in Yemen (A. M. Cohen, *American Heart Journal,* 1963),
- and entire countries such as Sweden, where the heart-disease death rate is only one-third of that in the U.S. (Werko).

Let's look at only one of these studies here—the Northern Indians compared to the Southern Indians. Dr. S. L. Malhotra (Chief Medical Officer, and Head of Medical Department, South Eastern Railway, Calcutta, India) compared railway sweepers of known constitution in identical trades and with identical amount of physical exercise, but with widely different intake of dietary fats. The Northern Indian railroad sweepers who regularly ate 10 times *more* fats derived from fresh milk or fermented milk showed 15 times *less* coronary heart disease than the Southern Indian railroad sweepers in similar socioeconomic levels, in the same age group of 18 to 55 years. In fact the very little fat that the Southern Indians did get was from the unsaturated fatty acids of seed oils. The Northern Indians even smoked 8 times more than the Southern Indians.

Dr. Malhotra remarked in a later article, "The cholesterol levels of both groups not only showed no statistically significant differences, but were low by Western standards. Thus, population groups with similar low serum cholesterol levels exhibited big differences in the incidence rates of coronary heart disease. Clearly levels of serum cholesterol do not play the crucial role ascribed to them and the evidence from the studies of others is in agreement with this view." (*American Journal of Clinical Nutrition*, 1971.)

Dietary Cholesterol Does Not Cause Heart Disease

There are scores of studies that show that cholesterol in the food does not cause heart disease. Unfortunately, these studies are complicated by the varying activity levels of the groups. The tests usually show that the group eating the most cholesterol has the lowest heart-disease death rate, but the persons in these groups are also usually more active, and thus may have had healthier arteries and burned up the extra fat and cholesterol.

One such study, the Ireland-Boston Heart Study, illustrates this point well. The study was jointly headed by Dr. Frederick J. Stare (of Harvard University's School of Public Health) and Dr. W. J. E. Jessop (of the School of Medicine of Trinity College, Dublin, Ireland).

A team of 19 researchers, including cardiologists and nutritionists, studied 575 pairs of brothers between the ages of 30 and 65. All brothers had been born and subsequently raised at least 20 years in Ireland. One of each pair of brothers had emigrated to the Boston area and lived there at least 10 years. Controls included another 312 urban and 152 rural Irishmen unrelated to the 575 pairs of brothers, plus 375 first-generation American men whose parents had been born in Ireland.

Both dietary and serum cholesterol were measured in addition to physical activity and body fat. The hearts of the participants were studied in detail and their diets were thoroughly evaluated. It was found that the hearts of the Irishmen were healthier and their blood pressure and serum cholesterol levels lower, even though their dietary cholesterol and calorie intake were higher. Their rich diets (lots of butter, milk, cream, bacon, potatoes, mutton, and brown bread) produced lower heart-disease rates.

Autopsies performed on participants who died during the study from accidents or noncardiovascular disease revealed that the hearts of the Irish brothers averaged 15 to 30 years younger than those of the American brothers. Generally, the Boston brothers developed lesions involving over 50 percent of the surface of the intima about 15 years earlier than those in Ireland. And, the Boston brothers ate more polyunsaturated fats (J. Brown et al, *World Review of Nutrition and Diet,* 12:1, 1970).

Activity and Lifestyle Are Related to Heart Disease

A series of studies of various occupational groups complement these findings. Studies among workers having the same diets, but different work activities, such as bus drivers/conductors, and mail clerks/postmen, showed that while the paired groups had similar cholesterol levels in their blood, the more active workers had fewer heart-disease deaths (J. N. Morris et al., *Lancet,* 1953; and H. A. Kahn, *American Journal of Public Health,* 1963).

Lifestyle is also related to heart disease. A nine-year study at the University of California at Berkeley of almost 4,000 Japanese-Americans living in California indicated that lifestyle has more significance than fat or cholesterol in the diet. They found that those Japanese-American men who maintained close ties to the traditional Japanese culture had a much lower rate of heart disease than those who shifted toward a more Western lifestyle.

They're Still Trying to Prove Cholesterol Is the Villain

There are two major studies running at present that have been touted as providing the answer about cholesterol and heart disease. They won't, however, provide the answer, because they are not designed to test cholesterol and heart disease in normal people. But if by chance the studies show what is expected, the anticholesterol people will have a field day proclaiming that they have proved cholesterol causes heart disease.

The largest study, nicknamed "Mr. Fit," which stands for Multiple Risk Factor Intervention Trial, involved screening 366,000 people at 20 clinical centers in the U.S. Of those screened, 12,500 men between 35 and 57 years old were selected who had three heart-disease risk factors: high blood cholesterol, high blood pressure, and a history of cigarette smoking. As you can see, these 12,500 people are not representative of the U.S. population.

The test is designed to determine whether heart-disease risk can be lowered—but it is not designed to find out what factors were responsible for lowering the risk. The test subjects will take medication to lower their blood pressure and medication to lower their blood cholesterol; they will eat fewer fats and cholesterol, reduce smoking, increase their physical activity, and receive excellent medical care. The planning for this study was initiated in 1972 and was described in the *Journal of the American Medical Association* in February 1976. The actual experiment will last six years (until 1980–81) and is expected to reduce heart disease deaths by 40 percent. If it does reduce heart disease deaths by even half that much, it will indicate helpful guidelines for those in similar circumstances. But it will not provide useful information about the necessity for low-cholesterol and low-fat diets among healthy persons.

Another important study is the Lipid Research Clinics Program, involving 4,000 men between the ages of 35 and 59. These men will be studied at 12 research centers to see if lowering the blood cholesterol levels with drugs and diet will reduce their likelihood of dying from heart disease.

All men in this study will have a genetic defect called hyperlipoproteinemia. This genetic defect occurs in about 1 out of 400 to 1 out of 1,000 people (they're not sure yet), and prevents normal cholesterol metabolism. Men with hyperlipoproteinemia have anywhere from 2.5 to 10 times the chance of dying of heart disease before the age of 50 as a "normal" person. Again the effect of drugs and diet on the individuals being tested may be beneficial. But that result will not mean that healthy individuals should restrict their diets accordingly—and the test results should not be so interpreted.

If you have a family history of early heart-disease deaths, make sure that during your annual physical exam you have a blood-chemistry test that includes phenotyping. This will determine whether you are one of those few individuals with one of the five genetic disorders called hyperlipoproteinemia. If you are, a dietary modification seems to be beneficial. Appendix 4 offers a summary of the dietary restrictions suggested by the Office of Heart Information, National Heart, Lung, and Blood Institute.

The gloomy prognosis for individuals with hyperlipoproteinemia is an exaggeration. In a recent angiographic study there was no difference in the severity of coronary heart disease between patients with hyperlipoproteinemia and those with normal values (Fuste, et al., *British Heart Journal,* 1975).

It has been found that a low-fat diet, including unsaturated fats, causes a drop in the blood cholesterol of 15 to 20 percent for about six to nine months, but that thereafter *cholesterol returns to previous values despite the diet* (Harlan, *Medicine,* 1966).

Unless you have hyperlipoproteinemia, eggs, meat, milk, and butter should be in your diet and can be eaten without fear. You can even eat fried foods and live longer. Dr. Harold J. Morowtiz of Yale University studied the health records of 422,000 men and found that the death rate for men who ate no fried foods at all was 72 percent higher than those who ate fried foods more than 15 times a week.

The important point, of course, is that you shouldn't live in fear of cholesterol. Relax, eat well, but watch your calories. Cholesterol doesn't count, but calories do.

6

Low-Cholesterol Diets
Don't Reduce Heart Disease

Pseudo-Scientific Organization Fronts for
Manufacturers of Polyunsaturated Oils

To date (1977), all attempts to reduce heart-disease deaths by lowering dietary cholesterol have failed. Often, in fact, such attempts have increased the heart-disease death rate. Unfortunately, there is actually a conspiracy by the polyunsaturated food manufacturers to perpetuate the cholesterol myth at the taxpayers' expense.

As just one example, the U.S. Government has given over $6 million of our tax money to a "front" for the polyunsaturated oil manufacturers, so that they may implement their goal of extensively changing the American diet by further increasing the sale of polyunsaturated oils. Specifically, this particular "front" is a pseudo-scientific organization misleadingly called the "American Health Foundation."

In 1973, Dr. Edward R. and Cathey Pinckney reported in *The Cholesterol Controversy* that "the Chairman of the Board of Trustees of the American Health Foundation, David J. Mahoney, is also the President of Norton Simon, Inc., the leading producer of cottonseed oil (Wesson Oil), which is pointedly advertised as polyunsaturated." The Pinckneys also pointed out that the position papers and the foundation's policy were formulated by Corn Products International (CPI—makers of Mazola margarine) executives Drs. Daniel Melnick and Dorothy Rathmann, who served on the foundation's Committee on Food and Nutrition. Perhaps in this case, health refers to the health of margarine sales and not of people.

In July 1972, the National Cancer Institute (a totally tax-supported organization) awarded this commercial foundation $2 million of tax money to further a program to prevent cancer and to assist in the construction of a new Health Research Institute. (Later in this chapter we will discuss two studies with some evidence that excess polyunsaturated fatty acids increase the cancer rate.)

In August of the same year, the National Heart, Lung, and Blood Institute (another thoroughly tax-supported organization) awarded the foundation $3.3 million of our tax money to research lowering elevated blood cholesterol. The thesis being tested was that increased polyunsaturate intake would lower serum cholesterol and by so doing reduce the risk of heart attack. Studies previously funded by the institute had showed that polyunsaturates did lower elevated blood cholesterol, but did not significantly alter morbidity or mortality.

In 1975, the NHLBI granted $1.1 million to the Mr. Fit program. It is interesting to note that the advisory steering committee for the Mr. Fit program includes two representatives from the American Health Foundation, Drs. Peter Peacock and Lloyd Shewchuk. In addition to the awarding of grants, the foundation spends a great deal of money in propaganda, including the publication of its own journal, *Preventive Medicine.*

When commercial organizations spend millions of dollars to convince the public of the health benefits of their food products, it's difficult to get the word across that those products do not yield the benefits their manufacturers claim. All too often in matters affecting health, it's not the best advice that gets the best press.

Another problem with the commercialism of the cholesterol controversy is regulation. Dr. Pinckney pointed out in his book that advertising and labeling of polyunsaturates may be misleading and not strongly enforced. I have complained several times to the FTC and FDA without as much as a polite (or even impolite) answer. One of the problems

may be seen here in the following quote from *The Choles-*
terol Controversy:

"In 1971 the general counsel for the FDA—the man in
charge of prosecuting any violations of FDA regulations (including those of mislabeled polyunsaturated products)—
left the FDA to become president of the Institute of Shorten-
ings and Edible Oils (the primary public relations group for
polyunsaturates). At the same time the man who had been
the legal representative of the edible oils companies suddenly became the general counsel of the FDA—the government lawyer now in charge of regulating and disciplining
the activities of his former clients."

It is illegal even to suggest that foods can be a medicine,
let alone cure heart disease. The following excerpts from
the *Federal Register,* Vol. 38, No. 13, Friday, January 19,
1973, make this perfectly clear:

**§1.18 Labeling of foods in relation to fat and fatty acid, and
cholesterol content.**

(a) Implicit or explicit claims for the value of food in preventing or treating heart or artery disease can be misleading to
consumers. However, a significant segment of the medical
community is recommending that individuals modify their total
diet by eliminating certain foods or by replacing certain foods
with others in order to effect changes in the levels of blood
components. Although there have been no definitive studies
which have demonstrated beyond doubt that extensive
changes in the consumption of fat and cholesterol by the general public are desirable, it is nevertheless appropriate to provide for informative labeling which will help individuals to identify foods for inclusion in fat-modified diets recommended by
physicans. It is also appropriate to prohibit label statements
which misrepresent specific foods as being, of themselves, of
value in the control of the levels of these blood components or
in the control of heart or artery disease.

(i) No label or labeling may contain a claim indicating, suggesting, or implying that the product will prevent, mitigate,
or cure heart or artery disease or any attendant condition.

The Prudent Low-Cholesterol Diet Group Had More Heart-Disease Deaths Than the Control Group

Although it has not been widely publicized, the test group following the first widely promoted low-cholesterol diet, the Prudent Diet, had more heart-disease deaths during a five-year experiment than the control group not following the low-cholesterol diet. In the control group (1,225 person-years) there were no deaths from heart disease, but in the low-cholesterol diet group (2,357 person-years), there were eight deaths from heart disease. More on the Prudent-type diets later, but first let's look at the recent studies of low-cholesterol diets and work our way back.

Studies in 1975 and 1976 Show No Relationship between Cholesterol Levels and Heart Disease

The Honolulu Heart Study of Hawaiian-Japanese men conducted in 1976 by a team of researchers headed by Dr. G. Rhoads (for the National Heart, Lung, and Blood Institute) investigated blood cholesterol levels and heart disease thoroughly. They found no relationship between total blood cholesterol levels and heart disease. They also examined the data from ten previous studies as reported in the scientific literature and concluded that these ten studies showed no relationship either.

A 1975 study of men in their 40s in Edinburgh and Stockholm showed that their blood cholesterol levels were within the same narrow higher-than-"normal" range, yet the Edinburgh men had three times the heart disease of the men in Stockholm (M.F. Oliver et al., *European Journal of Clinical Investigation,* 1975). Surely the higher-than-"normal" cholesterol levels couldn't be the primary cause of their heart disease.

The Minnesota Study concluded in 1975 involved 17,000 patients in state hospitals, where diets could be strictly controlled. Half the patients ate a normal diet, while the other half were given a diet lower in cholesterol and higher in unsaturated fats. After four and a half years, there were no significant differences in the number of heart attacks, strokes, and other cardiovascular problems between the two groups, although Dr. Ivan Frantz of the University of Minnesota reported "there were a few more events [heart attacks] in the treated than in the control group."

At the American Heart Association's annual scientific sessions in Anaheim, California, in 1975, Dr. Frantz reported that "despite a satisfactory decrease in blood cholesterol, there was not the slightest hint of benefit." (Polyunsaturated fatty acids can lower blood cholesterol levels by about 10 percent—but the cholesterol does not leave the body; it is only shifted to the liver and other depots.)

St. Vincent's Hospital Study Reveals the Risk of Overweight (1973)

What about those already having heart disease? Will lowering the blood cholesterol levels help them? Dr. M. L. Bierenbaum (of Saint Vincent's Hospital in Montclair, N.J.) sought to answer this question with a study begun in 1959.

In the study, 100 men initially between the ages of 20 and 50 and having confirmed myocardial infarctions were divided into two diet groups. Both diets were lower than normal in fats (28 percent vs. 40 percent lower). One diet contained one ounce of polyunsaturated oils (corn and safflower), thus providing a polyunsaturate-to-saturate ratio of 3 to 1, while the second diet contained one ounce of saturated oil (coconut or peanut), which yielded a polyunsaturate-to-saturate ratio of 1 to 3.

At the start of the study, many men were overweight, with the average overweight being 20.3 pounds. The overweight men in both groups were put on 1,200-calorie-per-day diets until their desired weight was achieved and maintained. (The reducing diets had the same polyunsaturate-to-saturate ratio as the test diets.) Both groups produced average cholesterol reductions of 10 percent.

The five-year follow-up was reported in the *Journal of the*

American Medical Association in 1967. At no time during the five years were there significant differences between the diet groups in serum cholesterol, triglycerides, incidence of recurring heart attacks, or mortality.

In the ten-year follow-up report, Dr. Bierenbaum concluded, "The degree of unsaturation of the diet did not appear to influence either serum lipid levels or mortality rates." (*Lancet,* 1973.)

An interesting observation about the test was made by Dr. William C. Sherman (Director of Nutrition Research for the National Live Stock and Meat Board): "After a year, when it was apparent that negative results would be obtained, a new 'control' group of 100 heart-attack survivors was recruited. They initially averaged 24.3 pounds overweight and none of them was reduced. They continued on their regular high-fat, high-calorie diet. After 5 and 10 years this 'control' group had approximately twice the incidences of recurring heart attacks and deaths as did the combined diet groups although no difference in serum cholesterol level was observed for the survivors and the deceased. *The trial indicated the harmful effects of prolonged obesity."* (*Food and Nutrition News,* 1976.)

Los Angeles Veterans Study Requires Careful Interpretation (1969)

A first look at the data from the eight-year study of 846 veterans at the Los Angeles Veterans Domicile merely indicates that the low-cholesterol diet had no effect on the heart-disease death rate. Closer inspection reveals some interesting observations. In the double-blind study by Drs. S. Dayton, M. L. Pierce, and colleagues, the veterans (many above the age of 70 and most of them hospitalized) were divided into two dietary groups. The control group received a diet in which 40 percent of the calories were mostly of animal origin, while the experimental group received a similar diet except that a mixture of vegetable oils replaced two-thirds of the animal fat.

The experimental diet (higher in vegetable oils) did lower serum cholesterol by nearly 13 percent, but the mortality from all causes in that group was slightly, although not significantly, higher (177 deaths in the experimental group vs. 174 in the control). The number of heart-disease deaths in the experimental (vegetable-oil) group was slightly, but not significantly, lower. However, the control group had more heavy smokers (70 vs. 45) and nearly twice as many veterans over 80 years of age (21 vs. 12). An analysis of these factors appearing in *Lancet* (in 1970) showed that the heavy smokers had more heart-disease deaths, which unbalanced the overall results. Dr. Sherman also pointed out in *Food and Nutrition News* that most of those over 80 died during the eight years of the study, and this again unbalanced the results.

If the study is adjusted to compensate for the unequal number of heavy smokers and older veterans in the control (animal-fat) diet group, the result is both fewer deaths of any type and fewer deaths due to heart disease for the group. It should be noted that there was a higher incidence of cancer in the experimental (vegetable-oil) diet group.

This study is one often used by the anticholesterol advocates to convince us to eat less cholesterol and saturated fats, but they never mention the cancer incidence, the heavy-smoker distribution, or the disproportionate number of older veterans eating the animal-fat diet.

Finnish Mental Hospital Study Reveals Possible Link between Low-Cholesterol Diets and Cancer (1968)

Another study often quoted by anticholesterol advocates is the 12-year Finnish Mental Hospital Study involving two mental hospitals in Helsinki. But it is highly likely that mismanagements of the diets administered distorted the results. Finland is the country with the greatest heart-disease rate, and the experiment was designed to have one hospital give a normal Finnish diet to its patients for six years, while the other provided a low-cholesterol, high-polyunsaturated-fatty-acid diet for its patients. After six years, the hospitals were supposed to switch diets for another six-year period.

Unfortunately, the experiment wasn't carried out that way. When the hospital that was first giving its patients the low-cholesterol diet switched to the normal Finnish diet, it supplied a diet so much heavier in calories than the other diets in the study that it produced an average gain of 40 pounds per patient during the following six-year experiment.

In the first six years of the study, when the calorie intake was kept at reasonable levels, the experimental cholesterol-lowering diet did reduce the average blood cholesterol levels by 10 percent. However, there were no significant differences between the two groups in either heart disease or total disease mortalities.

In the second part of this study, the difference that the high-calorie diet made was readily apparent. Although the number of deaths from all causes was essentially the same in both groups, the heart-disease death rate among the men receiving the extra calories was higher. It is quite possible that the small difference in heart-disease mortality was due to differences in calorie intake and obesity. The factor that kept the number of deaths from all causes equal in each group was the increase in cancer deaths among the patients on the low-cholesterol experimental diet.

London Medical Research Council Study Shows No Benefits from Polyunsaturates (1968)

One of the studies in which reducing saturates while increasing polyunsaturates proved to be of no benefit in treating survivors of heart attacks was the London Medical Research Council Study.

A group of 23 physicians from six London hospitals pooled their resources and for a four-year period studied 393 men under 60 years of age who had each had one heart attack. The men were divided into two groups. The control group ate a normal diet, with a polyunsaturate-to-saturate ratio (P/S) of 1 to 6. The P/S ratio was 2 to 1 in the experimental diet group, which eliminated all foods high in saturated fats and added three ounces of polyunsaturated soybean oil daily, half taken as a liquid supplement (which could have produced a beneficial placebo effect).

All overweight men in both groups were placed on reducing diets (with the same P/S ratio as the others of their group). The experimental high P/S ratio diet did reduce the blood cholesterol levels by 15 percent, whereas the normal diet produced only a slight lowering of the blood cholesterol. The weight reduction among the overweight in both groups contributed to the lowered cholesterol averages of both groups.

No significant differences could be found in heart-attack incidence, heart-disease death rate, or types of heart-disease relapses. The investigators concluded, "There is no evidence from the London Trial that the relapse rate in myocardial infarction is materially affected by the unsaturated fat content of the diet used." (*Lancet,* 1968)

National Diet Heart Study Shows No Benefits From Polyunsaturates (1968)

Researchers in five U.S. centers (Baltimore, Minneapolis–St. Paul, Oakland, Chicago, and Boston) studied 250 men aged 45 to 54 years in each city, some with and some without heart disease. Half were given polyunsaturated diets and half received control diets. Despite diet, the groups developed similar heart-disease records.

Norwegian Study Shows Benefits of Lower-Calorie Diets (1966)

Two years prior to the reports from the London Medical Research Council Study, rather similar results were published from a Norwegian study. The study included 412 men aged 30 to 64 years old who had survived their first heart attack.

Half of the men received an experimental diet which was low in animal fat, plus a special supplement (2.5 teaspoons of soybean oil and skim-milk powder taken daily) to give them twice as much polyunsaturated as saturated fats. The other half of the men continued their normal diet.

At the end of the study there was no difference in the death rate between those on the low-fat diet and those eating a normal diet (*Acta Medica Scandinavica,* 1966).

It is important to note that the experimental low-fat diet contained only 2,400 calories (compared to 3,000 calories in the normal diet) and produced an average weight loss of 5.5 pounds. Each group had 27 heart-disease deaths, although there were fewer heart attacks in the lower-calorie, experimental-diet group (43 vs. 64), and the men in the higher-calorie, standard-diet control group did experience an average increase in blood pressure. Perhaps the lower blood pressure and lower rate of heart attacks was due to the beneficial weight loss.

Anti-Coronary Club Demonstration Claimed Success but Produced Mixed Results (1966)

Earlier in this chapter, I mention the "Prudent Diet" developed by Dr. Norman Jolliffe (Director of the Nutrition Bureau of the New York City Health Department). Dr. Jolliffe, a well-liked nutritionist, was an expert in weight reduction and knew the value of weight control through personal experience with his own diabetes. He was clever in developing methods to help others lose those extra pounds, and published the book *Reduce and Stay Reduced* in 1952, followed by *The Reducing Diet Guide.*

In 1957 he started the Anti-Coronary Club to demonstrate that a diet that minimized several heart-disease risk factors would be prudent. He attacked obesity by restricting calories, high blood pressure by restricting salt, and high blood cholesterol by restricting fat and cholesterol.

The experimental group of 814 men between 40 and 59 years of age with no overt signs of heart disease were placed on a low-cholesterol, high-polyunsaturate diet having three units of polyunsaturates for every two units of saturates. Members of the group consumed at least 1 ounce of vegetable oil daily and only 1.6 grams of salt. They were given plenty of guidance and encouragement by the health officials, originally led by Dr. Jolliffe. The experimental group was further divided into an "active" group that attended regular meetings and had many tests, and an "inactive" group that followed the diet but did not attend meetings.

A control group of 463 men of the same age, also apparently free of heart disease, continued their normal diets, which had approximately three units of saturated fat for each unit of polyunsaturated fat. They were given no attention except for a yearly physical examination.

Unfortunately, Dr. Jolliffe passed away from vascular complications of diabetes at age 59; therefore, the five-year report was published by his colleagues. The report revealed that the prudent dieters had 8 coronary deaths (3 heart-disease deaths in the "active" group and 5 in the "inactive" group) while the control group eating the standard American diet had *no* fatalities due to heart disease.

There were fewer nonfatal heart attacks in the Prudent Diet group (8 per 2,357 man-years as opposed to 12 per 1,225 man-years). Perhaps this better showing was a result of this group's concentration on reducing obesity and high blood pressure. The control group made no such attempt to lower either factor. But as Wayne Martin, author of *Medical Heroes and Heretics* (Devin Adair Co., 1977), concluded, "So the founder of this study died of vascular complication, and there were 8 deaths from heart attacks in the experimental group as compared to none in the control group; and this was said to be 'successful medicine'!"

St. Mary's Hospital Study Reveals Corn Oil May Be Harmful to Those with Heart Disease (1965)

An earlier study by Dr. G. A. Rose (of St. Mary's Hospital) reported in the *British Journal of Medicine* in 1965 is very enlightening, but as you will see, will not be acknowledged by the polyunsaturate proponents.

Eighty male patients with a history of heart disease were given one of three diets with the same calorie content: a normal diet for the control group, and a low-animal-fat-plus-olive-oil diet or a low-animal-fat-plus-corn-oil diet for the experimental groups. The oils were given as 3-ounce liquid supplements each day.

At the end of the four-year study, 48 percent of those on the corn-oil diet had heart attacks; so had 43 percent of those on the olive-oil diet; but only 25 percent of the normal-diet group had heart attacks. There were twice as many serious heart attacks in the corn-oil group as in the control group. The investigators concluded, "Under the circumstances of this trial, corn oil cannot be recommended as a treatment for ischemic heart disease. It is most unlikely to be beneficial, and is possibly harmful."

London Research Committee Study Criticizes Low-Fat Diet (1965)

In that same year, a London study was published that reached the same conclusion: "A low-fat diet has no place in the treatment of myocardial infarction." (K. P. Ball et al., *Lancet,* 1965.)

In this three-year study, 264 male heart patients under 65 years of age were divided into two groups, one on a 2,000-calorie-per-day low-fat diet, the other group on a 2,400-calorie-per-day normal diet.

The low-fat diet did produce lower blood cholesterol levels and greater weight loss than the control diets, but the number of heart attacks and deaths combined was essentially the same (46 vs. 48 respectively).

And New Zealand agrees! In *Coronary Heart Disease,* Report of a Committee of the Royal Society of New Zealand (1971), primary emphasis was placed on nutritional and environmental factors. They critically reviewed all of the studies published by early 1971 and concluded that the key nutritional factor was total calories.

They concluded, "In particular, aggressive efforts to encourage the New Zealand population to increase the consumption of polyunsaturated fats at the expense of the present normal dietary fats are not justified."

American Cancer Society Study Demonstrated That Those Avoiding Eggs Developed More Heart Disease

What is the harm in avoiding cholesterol-rich eggs? For one thing, it's hard to achieve proper nourishment. Consider the study by Drs. Cuyler Hammond and Lawrence Garfinkel of the American Cancer Society which surveyed the diets of 800,000 Americans with no signs of heart disease. They divided the subjects into two groups and followed their health records for six years. One group consisted of those eating less than five eggs a week, the other those eating five or more eggs weekly. During the course of the study, those eating fewer eggs developed more heart disease. Results such as these are not discussed by the polyunsaturate adherents.

Physicians Disheartened by Failure of Low-Cholesterol Diets

Doctors are becoming dismayed at the failure of low-cholesterol diets to produce beneficial results. The secretary of the American Medical Association's Council on Foods, Dr. Philip L. White, told a 1974 meeting of food editors, "We are all tired by now of the unending advertisements for oils and margarines that promise to clear our arteries in much the same way a drain cleaner works."

Lowering blood cholesterol levels by dietary control hasn't prevented heart fatalities in any study yet published, and neither has lowering cholesterol with drugs, as you will see in the following chapter. Indications are that despite advertising claims to the contrary, you're better off eating eggs, milk, and animal fats than if you don't. This is because you get better nutrition. However, with care and vitamin and mineral supplementation, some low-cholesterol or low-fat diets can be beneficial if they are also low-calorie. The secret is to have a low-calorie, high-nutrition diet.

The Danger of High-Polyunsaturate Diets

The danger of polyunsaturates began to be noticed by Dr. Fred A. Kummerow and his colleagues from the University of Illinois at Urbana. When they reported their studies at the 1974 Federation of American Societies for Experimental Biology (FASEB) meeting of nutritionists and related sciences, newspapers carried the story under headlines such as "Margarine Found Health Hazard." Too bad the story didn't make the front sections. The findings showed that the trans-fats (manufactured hydrogenated fats) in margarine may present a real health hazard.

The studies involved feeding different types of diets to various groups of swine for eight months. (Swine were used in the tests because the aorta and heart of a pig weigh about the same as those of a human, and pigs are close to humans in their response to cholesterol.) The experiments were repeated several times with identical results. The greatest degree of hardening of the arteries was in the pigs fed margarine base stock with their diet. The group fed sugar with their diet was next. The group fed butter had almost negligible damage, and the least disease was found in the groups fed egg yolk or egg whites with their standard diet. (The degree of atherosclerosis developed as a result of the diet was determined by autopsies on the laboratory animals.)

The researchers concluded that hydrogenated fats (trans-fatty acids) which are contained in margarine base stock designed to make the product more stable were more atherogenic (plaque-causing) than cholesterol-rich foods such as butter and eggs.

It's not just margarines, but even egg-substitutes. One egg-substitute was tested by Dr. Kummerow and found to be lacking, if not downright dangerous. In his experiment, three separate groups of nursing rats had their diet of mother's milk supplemented by unlimited amounts of either egg-substitute, whole eggs, or lab chow. After one week the rats on the egg-substitute developed diarrhea. At three weeks the egg-substitute diet rats weighed only half as much as the other two groups. After two more weeks all the rats were weaned, and four weeks later, all of the rats on the egg-substitute diet were dead.

A similar study was made with chicks at the University of New Mexico. Chicks receiving the egg-substitute diet lost weight and were all dead after being on the diet for only 12 days. Chicks on eggs or starter mash suffered no fatalities even after three weeks, so the experiment was concluded.

Some Polyunsaturates Are Essential to Life

Some polyunsaturates (2–4 percent of the diet) are needed by the body, but an excess (greater than 10 percent) may be harmful.

Polyunsaturates are fats produced principally by vegetation. People and animals have polyunsaturates in all of their cells, and some quantity of three of the polyunsaturates (arachidonic acid, linoleic acid and linolenic acid) are needed regularly in the diet. Polyunsaturates are needed for cellular membrane health and the production of prostaglandins (hormonelike chemicals). They are important to growth, maintenance of skin and hair, regulation of cholesterol metabolism, maintenance of reproductive functions, and regulation of blood-platelet adhesion. Polyunsaturates are oils while saturates are solid fats. (Table 7.1 lists the percentage of saturation and polyunsaturation in several foods.)

The Recommended Daily Allowance of the Food and Nutrition Board (8th edition, 1974) is a polyunsaturate intake of 1–2 percent of total calories. However, many, if indeed not most, Americans are exceeding this recommended intake of polyunsaturates. Table 2.4 in Chapter 2 shows that the intake of polyunsaturates in 1963 was twice that of 1909. Dr. Pinckney estimated (in *Medical Counterpoint*) that in 1973 the average American ate between 4 and 6 percent polyunsaturates, which was two to three times the average consumed in 1950.

Table 7.1

Amount of Fats in Some Popular Foods. (Percentages Do Not Equal 100 Percent)

Food	Total Fat	Unsaturated	Saturated
Salad and Cooking Oils			
Safflower	100	87	10
Sunflower	100	84	11
Corn	100	81	13
Cottonseed	100	71	23
Soybean	100	75	14
Sesame	100	80	14
Peanut	100	76	18
Olive	100	83	11
Coconut	100	6	80
Vegetable Fats— shortening	100	46	23
Margarines— First ingredient on label			
Safflower, tub	80	66	11
Corn Oil, tub	80	64	14
Soybean oil, tub	80	64	15
Corn oil, stick	80	62	15
Soybean oil, stick	80	65	15
Cottonseed, partially hydrogenated	80	65	16
Butter	81	29	46

Table 7.1 (cont.)

Food	Total Fat	Unsaturated	Saturated
Animal Fats			
Poultry	100	60	30
Beef, lamb, pork	100	50	45
Fish, Raw			
Salmon	9	6	2
Mackerel	13	7	5
Herring, Pacific	13	5	4
Tuna	5	3	2
Nuts			
Walnuts, English	64	50	4
Walnuts, black	60	49	4
Brazil	67	49	13
Peanuts or peanut butter	51	39	9
Pecan	65	72	6
Egg Yolk	31	15	10
Avocado	16	9	3

Arthur L. Frank, *Bestways,* November 1975.

I do not agree with the recommendation of the American Heart Association and the Inter-Society Commission for Heart Disease Resources that up to 10 percent of our total calories should be polyunsaturates (*Nutrition Today,* 1974; and I.S. Wright et al., *Cardiovascular Diseases,* 1974).

Some Recommended Polyunsaturate Levels Are Dangerous

We often hear of the importance of increasing the ratio of polyunsaturates to saturates in the diet. Basically, increasing the P/S ratio implies that the total amount of fats in the diet should be kept nearly constant, or reduced, while the saturates should be reduced and the polyunsaturates increased.

A less preferred alternative is to add polyunsaturates to the present diet, thereby increasing the P/S ratio, but also increasing the total fat. There are some polyunsaturate proponents who feel the P/S ratio is more critical in the control of heart disease than the total amount of fat consumed.

To obtain the P/S ratio, the amount of polyunsaturates is divided by the amount of saturates. Thus, a ratio of one part polyunsaturates to two parts saturates may be expressed as a P/S of 0.5. The standard American diet before the stress on polyunsaturates probably had P/S ratios less than 0.3. The recommendation of the agencies suggesting that 10 percent of calories be polyunsaturates while total fats are kept to less than 35 percent yields a P/S of 0.4 or higher. Yet, there are those who suggest a P/S ratio as high as 1.5 or 2.0. This is excessive and potentially dangerous.

One of the reasons that a P/S of 1.5 to 2.0 is recommended is that polyunsaturates in the P/S range from 0.1 to 1.6 do not lower blood cholesterol levels (W.E. Connors et al., *Journal of Clinical Investigation,* 1969). Other researchers have found that polyunsaturates cannot lower blood cholesterol unless total dietary fats are less than 30 percent of total calories. Even then we must ask where the cholesterol goes and whether it is better or worse to have it there than to have it circulating freely in the bloodstream. Remember, the only harmful cholesterol is that which is produced *within* the plaque formed in diseased arteries.

Excess Polyunsaturates Have Been Linked to Cancer

The danger of excess polyunsaturates is in more than the fact that they drive cholesterol from the bloodstream into the liver and body cells. The prime danger is that excess polyunsaturates promote the release of free radicals and dienes. Free radicals (very reactive molecular fragments) are produced as the polyunsaturates react with oxygen in the body (in effect, to turn rancid in the process). Free radicals accelerate the aging process, cause cancer, and initiate the mutation process (monoclonal proliferation) that causes plaque to form in arteries. Dienes are the polyunsaturate fragments that can cause cellular damage as well as form free radicals. (See Appendix 3.)

The release of free radicals and dienes explains how *excess* polyunsaturates act as co-carcinogens in accelerating cancer formation. Optimal amounts of polyunsaturates (2–4 percent of calories) supply needed double-bond fats, but do not contribute more free radicals than can be handled by the free-radical absorbers or scavengers such as vitamin E and selenium. When greater amounts of polyunsaturates are consumed, the requirement for vitamin E and selenium is raised for several months after consumption, because the body prefers to store essential polyunsaturates rather than saturates, and because vitamin E is lost from the body much faster than polyunsaturates.

Corn oil, which is rich in polyunsaturates, has been reported by Dr. J. Szepsenwol to cause cancer in mice (*Proceedings of the American Association of Cancer Researchers,* 1971). In experiments with laboratory animals, several researchers have shown that excess polyunsaturates potentiate the tumor-inducing properties of other carcinogens (F. Bischoff, *Journal of the National Cancer Institute,* 1957; M. Sugai et al., *Cancer Research,* 1962; E. B. Gammal et al., *Cancer Research,* 1967; K. K. Carroll and H. T. Khor, *Cancer Research,* 1970; *Lipids,* 1971; R. Shamberger, *Journal of the National Cancer Institute,* 1972; C. E. West and T. G. Redgrave, *American Laboratory,* 1975; B. S. Mackie, *American Laboratory,* 1976).

To protect against excess polyunsaturates, be sure you get adequate amounts of the antioxidants vitamin E and selenium, plus biotin and vitamin B_{12} (DuPont and Matthias, *Lipids,* 1969) and vitamin A (Sherman, *Journal of Nutrition,* 1941).

Cancer is a major threat to life, yet the prime connection made between personal health and food advertising continues to focus on the mythical association of high polyunsaturates and reduced incidence of heart disease. The fact is, a far better case could be made by the producers of butter, milk, and eggs that high-polyunsaturate diets (including margarine, corn oil, non-dairy creamers, and egg substitutes) increase the incidence of heart disease and cancer. Besides animal experiments, which implicate diets high in polyunsaturates with the production of cancer-causing agents, the low-cholesterol diet experiment at the Los Angeles Veterans Hospital by Drs. Dayton and Pierce (detailed in Chapter 6) also revealed a higher incidence of cancer among those on the vegetable-oil diet.

This, of course, is not conclusive proof; but, since excess polyunsaturates do no good, and possibly much harm, I can't encourage the excessive use being promoted by mass advertising and misinformed physicians; and I have to speak out against the daily encouragement of advertisers to eat more and more polyunsaturates.

High-Polyunsaturate Diets Are Linked to Premature Aging

Dr. Edward R. Pinckney conducted a double-blind study which evaluated dietary polyunsaturates as a factor in premature aging and wrinkling of facial skin. He found that among those who deliberately consumed more than 10 percent of their calories as polyunsaturates, 78 percent showed marked clinical signs of premature aging (and, in addition, they looked much older than their chronological age). In this same group, 60 percent reported that they had at least one or more skin lesions removed because of suspected malignancy *after* having altered the fat content of their diet.

In contrast, among those who made no special effort to eat polyunsaturates (this group's average intake was approximately 5 percent of their diet), only 18 percent were judged to have outward signs of premature aging and only 8 percent reported the removal of any precancerous or cancerous lesions from their skin at any time in the past.

Dr. Pinckney concluded, "It would seem medically proper, then, to warn patients not to go overboard on polyunsaturates in spite of the constant nonmedical [commercial] and paramedical [health-agency] pressure now being brought upon them." (*American Heart Journal,* 1973.)

High-Polyunsaturate Intake Causes Still More Problems

Additionally, patients following the American Heart Association's printed diet, which suggests a 15 percent intake of polyunsaturates, experience a significant increase in uric acid in the blood (W.S. Wilson et al., *Journal of the American Medical Association,* 1971). Elevated uric-acid levels are a definite risk factor in heart disease (*Lancet,* 1969), and indicate destruction of cellular nucleoprotein.

Other problems due to excess polyunsaturates are iron-deficiency anemia, liver disease, intestinal damage and obstruction, amyloidosis (abnormal waxy deposits in tissues) and hypertension (E.R. Pinckney, 22nd Annual Minnesota Academy of Family Physician's Refresher, 1972). Another problem associated with excess polyunsaturates is the higher frequency and extent of gallstones (H.B. Lofland, Federation of American Societies for Experimental Biology, Atlantic City, N.J., 1975).

Lastly, two studies have shown that atherogenesis (formation of atherosclerosis) is enhanced, rather than retarded as claimed, as more polyunsaturates are ingested (D. Kritchevsky, *Medical Counterpoint,* 1969; and D. Harman, Annual Meeting of the Gerontological Society, 1972).

Heated Vegetable Oils May Be Harmful

Heated vegetable oils may have accelerated cancer-inducing properties compared with nonheated oils. However, this acceleration has been observed only when the oils were heated under laboratory conditions and not with actual samples from commercial restaurants (G. A. Nolen, *Journal of the American Oil Chemists Society,* 1972).

Dr. David Kritchevsky (of the Wistar Institute in Philadelphia) has shown that "heating a polyunsaturated fat (especially corn oil) to 200 degrees Fahrenheit for 15 minutes (far less than normal home cooking temperature and time) actually enhanced atherosclerosis in animals." (Edward Pinckney, *Medical Counterpoint,* 1969.)

When a fat or oil is heated and begins to smoke, the glycerol portion (rather than the fatty acid portion) is dehydrated and acrolein is formed. The polyunsaturates do not become saturated, as some had believed, but are no longer simple oils. They combine and form solids.

Dr. Pinckney reports that "when animals were fed heated polyunsaturates and heated butter to note the effect on their health, all of the animals given heated corn oil developed tumors. . . . In contrast, none of the animals fed heated butter developed tumors, and all survived."

The Dangerous Properties of Margarine

In the commercial preparation of margarine, polyunsaturates are partially converted into mono-unsaturates and saturates to protect the margarine from heat damage and oxidation as well as to improve its consistency. This is accomplished by adding hydrogen to the polyunsaturated molecules, thus increasing the saturation (the number of hydrogen atoms in the molecule). This hydrogenation process converts many natural cis-fatty acids into trans-fatty acids. The cis- forms occur abundantly in nature, but the trans- forms are bad guys that occur only about 5 to 8 percent of the time. Trans- forms of fatty acids have been linked to heart disease.

Stick margarine contains from 25 to 35 percent trans-fatty acids, tub margarine contains 15 to 25 percent, shortening 20 to 30 percent, salad oils 0 to 15 percent, and visible animal fats about 8 percent (*Dairy Council Digest,* 1975).

The trans- form does not seem to lower blood cholesterol, and has increased blood cholesterol levels in swine fed 40 percent trans-fatty acids (T. Mizuguchi et al., Federation of

American Societies for Experimental Biology, Atlantic City, N.J., 1974; and A. Vergroesen, *Proceedings of the Nutrition Society,* 1972).

Even the extraction of vegetable oils can alter nature's product. Dr. Ross Hall reports that industry's method of choice for extracting vegetable oils is to crush the vegetable, add solvent (gasoline, hexane, benzene, ethyl ether, carbon disulfide, carbon tetrachloride, or methylene chloride), remove the liquid, and boil off the solvent. Up to 100 parts per million of the solvent remains. Free fatty acids are removed with lye. Then the oils are deodorized by heating at 330° to 380° F for 12 hours. Finally BHT or another antioxidant is added (*Food for Nought,* Harper & Row, 1974).

From this product margarine is made. You can see that the original molecules have been greatly altered, and that margarine is completely unnatural. The corn oil used in experiments by scientists may or may not be the commercial product, but what you get for your food is rarely nature's finest.

8

Cholesterol-Lowering Drugs Are of Questionable Value

"Do those drugs that reduce blood levels of certain fatty substances—notably cholesterol and triglyceride—confer any protection against recurrent heart attacks or improve long-term survival among men who have previously experienced one or more acute heart attacks?

"Apparently not, according to findings reported from the National Heart, Lung, and Blood Institute's Coronary Drug Project at a press briefing held January 24, 1975" and sponsored by the National Institutes of Health.

The above is quoted directly from a Department of Health, Education, and Welfare news release, and it sums up the status (at the time of this writing) of drug effect on heart disease. I don't want to imply that there is no hope for an effective drug to cure or prevent heart disease. Drugs might work at different dosages under different conditions. After all, a drug that lowers cholesterol just might coincidentally lower the platelet-adhesion index, decrease the fibrinogen levels, or produce some other action that would be effective.

Drugs widely advocated for the lowering of blood cholesterol include clofibrate (Atromid-S), cholestyramine (Cuemid, Questran), and nicotinic acid (niacin, vitamin B_3). Other drugs occassionally prescribed are neomycin (mycifradin, Neobiotic), estrogens, dextrothyroxine (choloxin), norethindrone (Norlutate), and sitosterols (cytellin).

One should ask how these drugs lower cholesterol and whether that is a good thing to do. For example, blood cholesterol could conceivably be lowered by any of the following: blockage of production of cholesterol in the body, increased rate of consumption or excretion of cholesterol, reduction of the blood proteins that transport cholesterol, prevention of the absorption of dietary cholesterol, or forcing of the cholesterol from bloodstream into the liver.

Lowering Blood Cholesterol Can Be Dangerous

Unfortunately, the procedures to lower blood cholesterol are not without risk. Cholesterol is needed by every cell in the body, so reducing cholesterol production throughout the entire body might compromise organs not oversupplied with cholesterol. The same inherent risk runs with metabolizing (burning up) cholesterol nonselectively. There should be concern for the effects on the glands and organs involved.

Blocking the absorption of cholesterol from foods could also block the absorption of needed fat-soluble vitamins, fats, and other fatlike nutrients. Reducing the number of available protein transporters (lipoproteins) for cholesterol might unfavorably oversaturate the blood balance of cholesterol and other compounds carried by these transporters. Forcing the blood cholesterol into the liver or other tissues, including arteries, may do more harm than good. Still, a drug may be found that reduces only the cholesterol formed in the monoclonal plaques. That would be beneficial.

Coronary Drug Project Reveals Those Dangers

The Coronary Drug Project Research Group, headed by Dr. Jeremiah Stamler (of Northwestern University Medical School) in collaboration with 53 participating clinics, involved 8,341 coronary patients between 30 and 64 years of age and evaluated five cholesterol-lowering regimens. The drugs evaluated were clofibrate, dextrothyroxine, nicotinic acid (niacin), and estrogen at two dosage levels. Estrogen, a female sex hormone, is a cholesterol-lowering agent. Clofibrate (a substituted aliphatic acid), dextrothyroxine (an analog of one of the thyroid hormones), and nicotinic acid (vitamin B_3) reduce both cholesterol and triglycerides.

Each regimen was administered to about 1,100 patients, with 2,789 patients receiving standard medical management plus a placebo serving as a control. The follow-up period was five years, though more than half were followed up after six years or more. The tests began at various times starting in March 1966.

Three treatment regimens were dropped during the course of the study when it became apparent that they were of no positive value. The first to go was the high-estrogen regimen. It was discontinued in 1970 because (a) it was not improving survival rates and (b) patients on this regimen were suffering more nonfatal cardiovascular events (specifically, nonfatal heart attacks, pulmonary embolism, and thrombophlebitis) than were the patients in the control group.

Dextrothyroxine was dropped in late 1971 because of decreased survival rates. Instead of an anticipated drop of 24.4 percent in coronary heart disease, the test group experienced an 18.4 percent increase in cardiac death, thus missing the target by 42.8 percent (*Journal of the American Medical Association,* November 6, 1972). It is possible that lower starting dosages and screening out patients with histories of certain heart-rhythm disturbances would have produced a better record, but this remains to be proven.

The low-estrogen regimen was dropped in 1973 largely because of evidence that it increased the risk of thromboembolism without any compensatory improvement in survival rates.

The other two regimens, clofibrate and nicotinic acid, were continued throughout the study and showed no significant benefit in improving survival when compared with the placebo group's experience (*Journal of the American Medical Association,* January 27, 1975).

In terms of patient survival or reduction in risk from cardiovascular problems, the benefits of drug therapy were small. The clofibrate group had a mortality rate nearly the same as that of control groups and a somewhat *higher* incidence of nonfatal cardiovascular events such as new angina, intermittent claudication, venous pulmonary embolism, and arrhythmias. No subgroups of the study population were identified in which clofibrate showed clear benefit in regard to mortality. Yet it is estimated that $75 million is spent annually in America alone on clofibrate.

The nicotinic-acid group also had nearly the same mortality rate as that in the control group, a somewhat *lower* incidence of heart attacks, angina pectoris, and intermittent cerebral ischemic attacks, but a somewhat *higher* incidence of arrhythmias.

The study investigators concluded that "the Coronary Drug Project provides no evidence on which to recommend the use of clofibrate in the secondary prevention of coronary heart disease. . . . Nicotinic acid may be mildly beneficial in protecting persons to some degree against recurrent myocardial infarctions. However, because of the excess incidence of arrhythmias, gastrointestinal problems, and abnormal chemistry findings in the nicotinic acid group, much care and caution must be observed in the use of this drug."

By the way, another interesting fact arising out of this study is that more than half of the 8,341 men in the study, all of whom had suffered a heart attack, were found to have low blood cholesterol levels. This confirms what Dr. De-Bakey said in 1964 in the *Journal of the American Medical Association* (but no one listened).

Advertising of Cholesterol-Lowering Drugs Should Be Halted

Other drug studies where blood cholesterol level was lowered produced the same general results—no difference in mortality or a slightly poorer survival rate in the drug group (Oliver and Boyd, *Lancet,* 1961).

Of course, earlier studies involving smaller groups, such

as the United Airline Pilot Studies (*Journal of the American Medical Association,* 1972), had shown what appeared to be benefits in using the drugs, and the effect of drugs on men free of heart disease may be different.

Until medical research does come up with a drug that proves to be effective, physicians should be warned of the present lack of proof, and advertising should be halted on these drugs, as it misleads the physicians who can't keep up with the voluminous research literature and raises false hopes in the patient. More attention in the prevention of heart disease should be directed to the use of antioxidant nutrients and toward preventing the combination of proven risk factors.

9
The Most Important Protection—Vitamin E

Nearly everyone has heard that Vitamin E is supposed to cure heart disease. Claims and counterclaims have appeared in the scientific literature and the lay press, and many scientists cannot discuss the issue without getting emotionally involved. Some have even closed their minds to the issue and refuse to read the latest research on vitamin E's role in preventing and curing heart disease. Others have followed the recent reports with interest, but still find they haven't seen *conclusive* proof as yet. Many of these same scientists and physicians earlier jumped on the anticholesterol bandwagon without sufficient proof, and that may account for their present caution. Fortunately, enough scientists have an open mind and the fortitude to present papers explaining why the new evidence has caused them to become vitamin E advocates.

Dramatic new evidence is now available to show that vitamin E does indeed prevent and cure heart disease. Part of the new research is my own, and part comes from laboratories such as that of Dr. K. Korsan-Bengsten and colleagues in Sweden.

For over 30 years, Drs. Wilfrid and Evan Shute have achieved outstanding results in Canada in treating more than 40,000 cardiac patients (including many Americans) with vitamin E. The scientific literature contains numerous reports by physicians concerning cases in which heart disease has been cured with vitamin E. Although the procedures involved in the cures have been explained in detail, most physicians persist in believing that vitamin E's role in the cure has not been proven because double-blind studies (with untreated control subjects) have not been conducted. However, these physicians readily use aspirin and digitalis in their practice, although neither drug was subjected to a double-blind study prior to its widespread use. Some physicians who refused to accept the evidence of vitamin E's effectiveness pointed out that no acceptable mechanism explaining the vitamin's effectiveness had been offered. Yet, the mechanism for aspirin's action was uncovered only in the last few years, and the mechanism for digitalis is still a mystery.

Vitamin E Is Multifunctional

Vitamin E is a multifunctional compound. Its activity in preventing and curing heart disease is more a pharmacological than a nutritive function, although both functions are involved. Emotion enters the picture when nutritionists claim that we need only 15 to 50 international units (IU), and health researchers report that hundreds of IU are beneficial in protection against heart disease.

Here's why their opinions differ. Nutritionists study healthy laboratory animals that are fed diets with varying degrees of vitamin E deficiency. The laboratory animals are then examined to see what level of vitamin E is required to keep the animals healthy. The health researchers, on the other hand, study a disease pathway and the effect that specific amounts of vitamin E have on the disease. Since most people past the age of forty have some degree of atherosclerosis, it is wiser for most people to take the amounts of vitamin E suggested by health researchers.

Tocopherol is the chemical name for vitamin E, the name that health researchers use, and I believe that name is preferable because its definition does not limit the function of the compound to only its nutrient usage.

Our bodies are free to use tocopherol in a variety of ways, wherever there is a need. In the case of atherosclerosis, there is a need for the pharmacological action. Because atherosclerosis is an abnormal condition, it is only when this abnormality is present that the corrective function of tocopherol can be observed. Thus, when it comes to understanding the effectiveness of vitamin E in curing heart disease, we should listen, not to nutritionists, but to health researchers and the physicians concerned.

The Many Ways Vitamin E Protects Us from Heart Disease

The pioneers in treating heart disease with tocopherol, Drs. Wilfrid and Evan Shute, attribute its effectiveness to six major points, each established as a result of their laboratory experiments and later confirmed by the laboratory experiments of others:

1) Tocopherol is an anticlotting agent that helps prevent blood clots in arteries and veins.
2) Tocopherol helps dissolve existing blood clots.
3) Tocopherol increases the blood's supply of available oxygen by improving the transportation of oxygen by the red blood cells.
4) Tocopherol reduces the need of the heart for oxygen by making the heart become a more efficient pump.
5) Tocopherol prevents undesirable excessive scarring of the heart after an infarct, and promotes a strong "patch" scar during the healing process.
6) Tocopherol is a vasodilator (at least of capillaries) and improves capillary permeability (the capacity to permit substances such as nutrients to enter).

Many additional facts about tocopherol have since been discovered. However, not all proven abilities of tocopherol that might be expected to combat heart disease are necessarily significant factors in the cure of heart disease, no matter how logical that seems. The only way to know if tocopherol is effective is to study its effect on people with and without heart disease. This I have done with the conclusion that tocopherol is highly effective. But before we examine the evidence from my studies, let's look at the major milestones discovered through the years.

In 1942 Drs. O. B. Houchin and H. A. Mattill published three studies of the effect of tocopherol on oxygen-deficient muscle tissues (two in the *Journal of Biological Chemistry* and one in the *Proceedings of the Society for Experimental Biology and Medicine*). As they explained in the articles, muscles in tocopherol-deficient animals have an oxygen consumption much above normal. Feeding tocopherol to these animals returns their oxygen-consumption rates to normal in ten to twenty-seven hours. The tocopherol, in fact, decreases the need for oxygen by 60 to 71 percent.

If your heart is being starved of oxygen because its arteries are partially blocked, it doesn't help to have poor oxygen efficiency. Tocopherol reduces the need for oxygen and increases your chance for survival. Athletes have known of the oxygen-sparing property of tocopherol for a long time and take such supplements regularly. And racehorse trainers have been giving tocopherol to race horses for just as long.

You may note that tocopherol plays a role similar to that of exercise. By proper exercise, you increase your cardiovascular-pulmonary efficiency and, consequently, you utilize oxygen more efficiently. (Exercise also increases your chances of surviving a heart attack.)

Tocopherol and exercise have another effect in common. They both encourage the establishment of additional blood vessels and dilate smaller blood vessels when there is an oxygen demand. This brings more blood to every part of the body and reduces the damage done by the blockage of any single vessel. Again, your chances of surviving a heart attack are increased.

Dr. M. Fedelsova (of the Faculty of Medicine at the University of Manitoba) showed that tocopherol deficiency produces marked abnormalities in heart metabolism, due to changes in both energy conduction and utilization (*Canadian Journal of Physiology and Pharmacology,* 1971).

Vitamin E Keeps Your Heart Younger

Dr. E. Cheraskin (Professor and Chairman, Department of Oral Medicine, University of Alabama Medical Center) and Dr. W. M. Ringsdorf, Jr. (Associate Professor at the same institution) explicitly detail evidence that the supposed inevitable increase of cardiovascular symptoms and signs due to advancing age can be thwarted by tocopherol. Their examination of the relationship between age and reported cardiovascular findings in both men and women shows that the increase in clinical symptoms paralleled age only in the subjects (80 percent of the total group studied) consuming less than the recommended dietary allowance (RDA) for vitamin E. They conclude: "A review of the clinical change during the experimental year revealed that the decrease in cardiovascular findings occurred only in the group of subjects characterized by an increase in the daily intake of vitamin E."

Further analysis of the data by Drs. Cheraskin and Ringsdorf showed that those receiving more vitamin E and better all-around nutrition had improved electrocardiograms, blood triglyceride levels lowered by half, and their number of clinical complaints decreased from an average of seventeen to an average of twelve. Dr. Cheraskin observed that "within the one-year period, the clinical picture of the group improved approximately 30 percent. Specifically, the average fifty-year-old had become more like a forty-year-old within twelve months. It is most exciting to consider the possibility of diminishing, rather than increasing, complaints as we grow older. Particularly thrilling is the potential of accomplishing this goal by relatively simple dietary means." The details were published in *Nutrition Report International* in 1970.

According to the *Wall Street Journal* (March 13, 1973), clinical trials in Mexico showed a reduction of angina pectoris with a combination of tocopherol and selenium. Essentially the same formula has been used successfully for angina pectoris in animals by veterinarians for more than ten years. (Both drugs are manufactured by a division of Chromalloy.)

Dr. James P. Isaacs of Johns Hopkins treated 25 patients with severe heart disease for ten years, prescribing daily supplements of tocopherol, vitamin C, zinc, manganese, and copper along with estrogen and thyroid hormones. During that period, only 2 of the patients died, rather than the 13 or more who would have been expected to die in that length of time. Dr. Isaacs has treated another group of 100 patients who completed the ten-year period in 1976, but results were not available at the time of this writing.

Vitamin E Is Effective in the Treatment of Angina

Dr. W. M. Toone reported that 400 IU of tocopherol given four times daily reduced the need for nitroglycerin treatment of angina pectoris in a significant number of patients. He performed a single-blind test with two groups of eleven patients. Four patients in the tocopherol group were able to reduce their nitroglycerin use to two tablets or fewer per month; no patients in the placebo group reduced their use of nitroglycerin to fewer than eighty tablets per month (*New England Journal of Medicine,* 1973).

Vitamin E Prevents Blood Clots

As early as 1949, Dr. Alton Ochsner, one of our most famed surgeons, reported in *Surgery* that "Vitamin E is an efficient anti-thrombic [anticlotting] agent, and is probably one of the principal anti-thrombins in the blood. By supplying anti-thrombin in the form of vitamin E, the deficiency in anti-thrombin is corrected and a clot is prevented. The great advantage of using vitamin E is that although the thrombosing tendency is overcome, a hemorrhagic [bleeding] tendency is not produced, such as occurs when anticoagulants, for instance, heparin or dicumarol, are used."

Those anticoagulants (still commonly prescribed today) directly interfere with one factor of the clotting mechanism, and this interference is continuous and is not balanced by the other factors. Patients receiving those drugs for treatment of heart disease should be constantly monitored to see that their clotting time is not unnaturally prolonged, or they may bleed to death. **(Patients already on anticoagulants should not begin or change their tocopherol intake without notifying their physicians, as the tocopherol may change the coagulation time.)**

The year following Dr. Ochsner's first report, Dr. J. H. Kay and his Tulane colleagues verified the anti-thrombic effect, concluding that tocopherol combines with fibrinogen to form a complex that is not clottable with thrombin (*Proceedings of the Society for Experimental Biology and Medicine,* 1950).

In 1974, Drs. J. J. Corrigan and F. I. Marcus published a report that 800 IU of tocopherol taken daily caused a marked increase in prothrombin (clotting) time in a patient being treated with warfarin and clofibrate. In 1975, Dr. Corrigan confirmed the above (*Journal of the American Medical Association,* 1975), as did Drs. H. M. Soloman and J. Schrogie (*Journal of the American Medical Association,* 1975).

Blood Platelets Are the Key Factor in Preventing Blood Clots

The role of tocopherol in preventing heart-disease deaths is to reduce the stickiness of the blood, so that clots won't form. In 1972, a series of reports from Sweden noted that patients who had recovered from myocardial infarctions had a shorter plasma clotting time (stickier blood) than a population sample of the same size and sex. In 1974, the same group of investigators (Drs. K. Korsan-Bengsten, D. Elmfeldt, and T. Holm) published a paper reporting that patients taking 300 IU of tocopherol daily experienced improved clotting time and reduced their platelet adhesion after only six weeks (*Lancet,* 1975; *Thrombosis Diathes. Haemorrh.,* 1972, 1974; *Circulation,* 1970).

In 1975, Drs. P. M. Farrell and J. W. Willison, researchers for the National Institute of Health (NIH), reported at the Federation of American Societies of Experimental Biology

(FASEB) that large amounts of tocopherol may reduce platelet aggregation (blood stickiness and clotting). They observed that platelet counts were slightly lower in one-third of those taking between 100 and 800 IU of tocopherol daily.

In 1975, Dr. L. J. Machlin of Hoffman–La Roche observed markedly reduced platelet aggregation in laboratory rats fed extra tocopherol. Also the platelet count, which was higher in tocopherol-deficient rats, normalized when they were fed adequate tocopherol. Dr. Machlin's studies on platelet aggregation in laboratory animals were confirmed for humans by Dr. Manfred Steiner of Brown University (American Clinical Nutrition meeting, May 1976).

Also since my Survey Report (explained in the following chapter), Dr. Steiner and colleague John Anastasi (of both Brown University and The Memorial Hospital in Pawtucket, R.I.) published an interesting report in the *Journal of Clinical Investigation* (March 1976) concerning tocopherol and platelet adhesion. They found that platelet adhesion was reduced as the dosage of tocopherol was increased up to a level of 1,800 IU. In the men and women tested, platelet adhesion was reduced by up to 50 percent.

Platelets are plate-shaped blood components (less than half the size of red blood cells) that initiate blood clotting by forming a "clump" to which fibrin can adhere. Platelets especially adhere to the collagen produced in monoclonal smooth muscle cells growing in the arteries

The blood-platelet adhesion index is one of the major variables in heart disease. This index measures the clumping tendency, or "stickiness," of blood, through a measurement system in which normal blood is rated as 20–35. People who have just experienced a coronary thrombosis have platelet-adhesion indices over 90, and coronary-prone individuals have an index of 50 or greater. (The index number refers to the percentage of platelets that will stick to glass beads.) The number of platelets in a cubic millimeter of blood is about 200,000. (There are 16,387 cubic millimeters to the cubic inch.) The stickiness of the platelets can change without a change in platelet number.

Also keep in mind that tocopherol normalizes platelets in

such a manner as to reduce the release of factors (from the platelets) that stimulate monoclonal proliferation. Thus tocopherol's action on blood platelets is to reduce clotting and reduce the platelets' action in causing plaques.

Birth-control pills and smoking both tend to increase the platelet-adhesion index. In fact, many of the side effects of oral contraceptive drugs resemble those resulting from vitamin E deficiency. Drs. L. Aftergood and R. B. Alfin-Slater (both of the School of Public Health, U.C.L.A.) have found that oral contraceptives decrease the blood level of tocopherol (*Lipids,* 1974).

Incidentally, diabetics have abnormal platelets that are uncommonly sensitive to aggregating agents. This may explain why diabetics are normally prone to heart disease.

Anticoagulant Drugs Are Ineffective against Platelet Clots

Anticoagulant drugs have no effect on the platelet-adhesion index, since anticoagulants interfere with clotting at a late stage, not at the platelet stage. However, platelet clot alone is sufficient to cause death. The effectiveness of tocopherol as compared to the ineffectiveness of anticoagulants in curing heart disease is explained by the fact that tocopherol affects the platelet stage.

An individual could have atherosclerosis to the point of extreme artery narrowing and rupture of the inner artery lining, and yet not have a heart attack because tocopherol kept the platelet-adhesion index normal, preventing a clot from forming. This is why taking tocopherol is the most important step in preventing heart attacks.

Other factors that normalize platelet-adhesion indices are garlic (Bordia and Bansal, *Lancet,* 1973) and the polyunsaturated fatty acid called linolenic acid (cis isomer) (*American Journal of Clinical Nutrition,* June 1975). While some linolenic acid is required in the diet, excesses could be harmful. (See Chapter 7.)

Vitamin E Lowers Blood Pressure

OK, it's clear that tocopherol plays a major role in preventing coronaries by keeping the blood platelets "slippery" and thus free-flowing, preventing the plaque from forming. In addition, tocopherol has been shown to have beneficial effects on high blood pressure.

Japanese researchers at the School of Medicine of Tokyo University, Dr. C. Naito and R. Sugawara, found that tocopherol significantly reduced the plasma lipoperoxides in cardiovascular patients with high blood pressure, causing the blood pressure to normalize.

Tocopherol Is More Than a Vitamin

The action of tocopherol in reducing platelet adhesion has been proven, but the action of tocopherol in preventing the monoclonal plaques of atherosclerosis has not been fully established. There is strong evidence, however, that tocopherol protects the cellular membranes against the mutagenic chemicals and free radicals that cause the cells to proliferate. Thus, adequate nutritional levels of tocopherol (as a result of its vitamin function) protect the artery cells from damage that can lead to atherosclerosis, while extra amounts of tocopherol (as a result of its pharmacological function) deactivate the free radicals. It is very likely that a vitamin E deficiency increases the probability for membrane damage resulting in cell proliferation.

Well, so much for explanations; now let's look at the results of my survey, explained in the next chapter.

10

Evidence That Vitamin E Actually Prevents Heart Attacks

Research explaining how tocopherol prevents heart disease is important, but the final proof is in testing a large number of people taking tocopherol to see if their hearts are healthier than the hearts of those not taking it. This is what I did in 1974 and 1975. The results were published in *Prevention* in the January to May and July to September 1976 issues.

I studied reports from 17,884 people between the ages of 50 and 98 years (nearly equally balanced between sexes) of whom 3,725 had heart disease. I discovered two important facts.

First of all, more than 80 percent of those with heart disease reported that tocopherol helped the condition measurably. People requiring 18 or more nitroglycerin pills for their angina reported they threw their nitroglycerin pills away within a month or two after starting tocopherol. Many reported that angina pains would return in a few weeks or months if they discontinued tocopherol, but would disappear once again soon after they resumed taking tocopherol.

It is possible that psychological factors could account for the improvement, but results of studies show that any placebo effect is small. And it is doubtful that the prevention of a heart attack can be greatly influenced by the placebo effect.

The second major finding of the survey was that tocopherol apparently prevents heart disease. It was notable that the amount of heart disease in any age group decreased proportionally with the length of time that tocopherol had been taken. In fact, the length of time was more important than dosage after a minimum level of 400 IU daily was reached.

Two Groups Show Lower Heart-Disease Incidence with Vitamin E

Two groups were especially interesting. One group consisted of those who had taken 400 IU or more of tocopherol daily for 10 years or more. The survey included 2,508 such

Figure 10.1 There is a strong correlation between length of time taking vitamin E and freedom from heart disease in all age groups responding to survey.

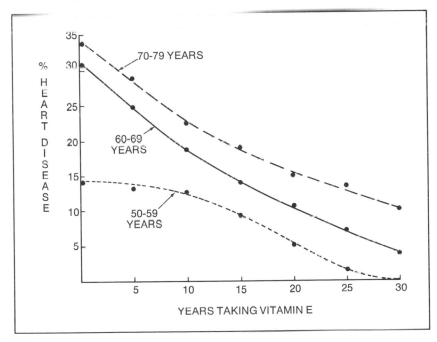

people between the ages of 50 and 98. Normally, based on the U.S. Dept. of Health, Education, and Welfare figures (HRS 74–1222), you would expect to find 836 of the 2,508 having heart disease. Instead there were only 4. This is less than one-half of 1 percent of the expected number.

A second group of 1,038 had taken 1,200 IU or more of tocopherol daily for 4 years or more. Among this group, you would expect to find 323 suffering from heart disease. But the actual number was 7.

A survey does not prove cause and effect. It only shows association, yet tocopherol was shown to be strongly associated with reduced incidence of heart disease.

The conclusions and projections that I have determined from the study are shown in tables 10.1, 10.2, and 10.3.

Still, few physicians will be convinced by either the findings of the survey or the early evidence from the 1940s and 1950s. However, the general population has found out for itself that tocopherol is effective.

The use of tocopherol tripled from 1970 to 1971, correlating well with the reports that heart-disease deaths in two age groups (45–54 and 55–64) have decreased by as much as 15 percent since that time through 1976.

Warnings for Those on Medication

Some people with high blood pressure or rheumatic heart disease may initially respond to tocopherol with an increase in pressure before it is lowered to normal. Therefore, they should begin any supplement only under their doctor's direct supervision and slowly (that is, with 50 IU daily the first month, increased by 50 IU each month until relief is found, generally around 800–1,200 IU daily). Blood pressure should be checked each month before increasing dosage.

For those on medication, tocopherol may reduce the amount of medicine required. If you are taking insulin, for example, the amount that you are taking might, with the tocopherol supplement, lead to insulin shock. Diabetics

Table 10.1

Heart Disease Incidence among Those Taking 400 IU of Vitamin E or More for 10 Years or More

Age Group	Number in Group	Expected Number with Heart Disease (National Rate from HEW Figures)	Actual Reported Number with Heart Disease (Possible Undetected Cases in Parentheses)		Percentage of Expected Number with Heart Disease
50–59	569	114	0	(3)	0
60–69	871	279	3	(1)	1.1
70–79	806	323	1	(2)	0.3
80–89	245	111	0	(1)	0
90–98	17	9	0	(0)	0
total	2,508	836	4	(7)	0.5

400 IU or more of vitamin E taken for 10 years or more is strongly associated with reduction of the incidence of heart disease prior to 80 years of age to less than 10 percent of the present rate (32 per 100 people expected to have heart disease reduced to 3 per 100 people who actually do have heart disease). Table 10.1 gives the data for this finding.

Table 10.2

Heart Disease Incidence among Those Taking 1,200 IU of Vitamin E or More for 4 Years or More

Age Group	Number in Group	Expected Number with Heart Disease (National Rate from HEW Figures)	Actual Reported Number with Heart Disease (Possible Undetected Cases in Parentheses)	Percentage of Expected Number with Heart Disease
90–98	1	0	0 (0)	—
80–89	64	28	0 (0)	0
70–79	284	114	2 (2)	1.8
60–69	356	114	4 (3)	3.5
50–59	333	67	1 (2)	1.5
	1,038	323	7 (7)	2.2

1200 IU or more of vitamin E taken for 4 years or more is strongly associated with reducing the incidence of heart disease prior to 80 years of age from 32 per 100 people to 10 per 100 people. Table 10.2 gives the data for this finding.

Table 10.3

Correlation Between Length of Time Taking Vitamin E and Freedom from Heart Disease

Years of Use of Vitamin E	Percentage Free from Heart Disease								
	0	Less than 1	1–3	4–5	6–9	10–19	20–29	30+	AVG.
Age Group									
50–59	85.7	86.6	86.1	86.2	86.7	89.2	98.3	100	86.8
60–69	68.4	69.6	73.0	74.9	78.7	85.5	89.1	100	76.1
70–79	67.8	64.6	69.1	71.0	70.7	82.1	81.8	88.5	73.6
80–89	65.2	71.8	69.3	67.5	66.9	81.2	85.6	00	73.3
90–98	87.5	100	94.8	77.8	91.7	96.8	—	00	93.4

The association between length of time taking vitamin E and freedom of heart disease is extremely strong statistically. The association (Spearman–Rho) is, in fact, stronger for vitamin E than any other tested variables, which included exercise, diet, and cholesterol intake. The association varies slightly with age,

but typically shows a 0.96 association where 1.00 is a perfect association. This correlation is significantly different from chance occurrence at the 0.01 level. Table 10.3 gives the data for this finding, and further data are given in Appendix 5.

Eighty percent of those with angina pectoris, fibrillation, or tachycardia are substantially helped by tocopherol within the first year of use. Most patients find

that they can gradually reduce other medication with increasing time and dosage of vitamin E.

on insulin should thus take vitamin E only under their doctor's close supervision.

Heart patients taking blood-thinners or anticoagulants must be checked monthly by their doctor to see if their blood becomes too thin or fails to clot for healing. They, too, should take vitamin E only under their doctor's direct supervision.

People allergic to wheat products, vegetable oils, or vitamin E should not take vitamin E supplements. However, they might try a 50 IU capsule to determine whether it is simply a particular form or brand that they are allergic to. Some will find that certain forms and brands may disagree with them, while others will not.

Researchers, Once Skeptical, Now See Value of Vitamin E

Researchers once skeptical about tocopherol's value in preventing heart disease are now changing their tune. The change isn't always abrupt, but the trend is obvious. As an example, consider the honesty and open-mindedness of Dr. M. K. Horwitt (of the Department of Biochemistry of the St. Louis University School of Medicine). During the Vitamin Information Bureau seminar held in Chicago in 1975, he remarked, "At this point in this interpretive paper, it is necessary for this long-time member of the nutritional establishment to eat some crow. For many years, suggestions that vitamin E might have an effect which might be useful in preventing circulatory disorders were dismissed with the comment that there is no evidence to justify such therapy. It must now be admitted that . . . there is a case for supporting the use of vitamin E as an antithrombic agent."

Dr. Horwitt went on to confess, "Nutritional scientists like myself have barely tolerated those who take supplements of vitamin E." But now he moderates his views. "Some of these claims which did not seem to have any credibility may now be more acceptable."

Now it's up to the medical profession to discover vitamin

E and its lifesaving properties. In the meantime, you can enjoy the protection it offers.

I have received (actually) thousands of letters from people telling me how tocopherol has helped relieve their heart trouble. To know how much you should take consult the final chapter, which presents the Supernutrition Program (which is a major factor in the Total Protection Plan).

In this and the preceeding chapter, I have presented some of the evidence that tocopherol prevents heart disease. It is the best preventive action that you can take, but it alone does not provide protection. Its best partner, the trace mineral selenium, is discussed in the next chapter.

11

Selenium–The Protector

The most exciting news in nutrition in the last ten years has been made by the micro-trace element selenium, an amazing mineral that helps protect human cells from cancer, heart disease, and premature aging. Laboratory research I conducted several years ago showed that selenium was a key ingredient in formulations that prevented cancer from occurring in experimental animals which had been exposed to known carcinogens. In other tests I conducted, selenium increased the lifespans of mice by slowing the aging process.

Selenium Protects against Heart Disease

Selenium has been recognized as an essential nutrient only since 1957, and its first known actual use by the body was not detailed until 1973. Since then, research interest has awakened.

Like iodine, selenium is not uniformly distributed in our soil, and consequently our food supply is apt to be deficient. (See Figure 11.1.)

At the 1976 Annual meeting of FASEB, Drs. Charles J. Shamberger and Charles E. Willis (of Cleveland Clinic) reported that Americans living in selenium-deficient areas are three times more likely to die from heart disease than those living in selenium-rich areas. Shamberger and Willis showed that the heart-disease rate in the 55-to-64-year-old age group was lowest in the selenium-rich states: Texas, Oklahoma, Arizona, Colorado, Louisiana, Utah, Alabama,

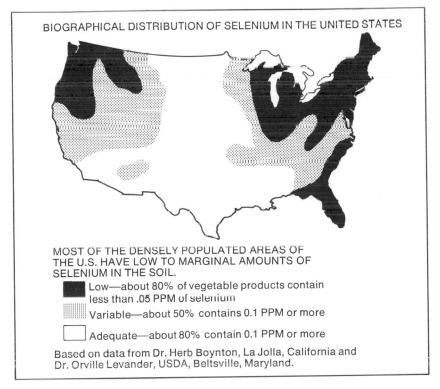

Figure 11.1 Most of the densely populated areas of the U. S. have low to marginal amounts of selenium in the soil.

Nebraska, and Kansas. At the top of the list of selenium-rich cities were Colorado Springs, Colorado, 67 percent below the national average for heart-disease deaths, and Austin, Texas, 53 percent below.

Unfortunately, most densely populated areas in the United States are deficient in selenium. But part of the exciting news about selenium is that selenium supplements are now available to correct selenium deficiencies (in the manner that iodized salt corrects iodine deficiencies in the goiter belt). More on selenium supplements toward the end of the chapter.

Although the nonuniform distribution is bad for the people living in the selenium-deficient areas, it's good for scientists studying selenium's protective effect against cancer and heart disease. It's relatively easy to compare the heart-disease incidence in areas deficient in selenium with those having adequate levels.

The selenium-deficient states, which according to the Shamberger-Willis studies include Connecticut, Illinois, Ohio, Oregon, Massachusetts, Rhode Island, New York, Pennsylvania, Indiana, and Delaware, produce a heart-disease death rate substantially higher than the national average. In the selenium-deficient District of Columbia, the heart-disease death rate during the years studied was 22 percent above the national average.

Of course, epidemiological studies show only association, not proof of cause and effect. But there is a lot of animal research to indicate cause and effect. For example, selenium has been studied with great interest by animal nutritionists and veterinarians, who have discovered that pigs, calves, and lambs fed selenium-deficient diets develop abnormal electrocardiograms, damaged hearts, and elevated blood pressure.

Selenium Normalizes Blood Pressure

In Chapter 9, I described how vitamin E protected against death from heart disease by several means including its functions in antioxidation, blood-pressure normalization, and normalization of the blood-platelet adhesion index. Selenium is similar to vitamin E in its effects and often acts as a partner with vitamin E. Both vitamin E and selenium are ambogenic, which means that both nutrients must be present to correct for a deficiency of either. The functions of vitamin E and selenium have three relationships: 1) one nutrient can substitute for the other for some, but not all, functions; 2) both nutrients are required to act together for a few functions; and 3) each nutrient has independent functions.

Blood-pressure normalization is a function of both nutrients which act together to control prostaglandins (a family of chemical messengers much like hormones, which control many bodily functions).

Dr. J. E. Vincent (of the Department of Pharmacology at the Erasmus University, Rotterdam, the Netherlands) believes that a selenium deficiency results in the inability to produce certain prostaglandins which, in turn, creates high blood pressure and the accumulation of a chemical intermediate in the arteries. The intermediate (a compound which accumulates because a selenium-containing enzyme is not available to incorporate it into prostaglandins) induces degeneration of the arteries and induces platelet aggregation (*Prostaglandins,* 1974).

Furthermore, Dr. Shamberger has found that selenium partly detoxifies (neutralizes) the adverse effect of the mineral cadmium, which induces high blood pressure in laboratory animals. As might be expected, areas containing high amounts of cadmium have higher than normal heart-disease death rates.

Selenium Protects against Plaque Formation

Selenium is a component of the enzyme glutathione peroxidase, which inhibits the aberrant oxidations that damage cellular membranes. Like vitamin E, selenium is required to protect cellular membranes against attack by free radicals and chemical mutagens that could cause the cell to proliferate wildly and cause plaque formation.

As noted in Chapter 9, vitamin E helped cure the clinical symptoms of 80 percent of those with angina and, when taken for several years, greatly reduced the incidence of heart disease. It well may be that the reason that 100 percent cure or protection was not achieved was that the unaffected cases were selenium-deficient.

Dr. L. H. Sprinker (of the Department of Veterinary Medicine of Oregon State University) and his colleagues reported (*Nutritional Reports International,* 1971) that selenium deficiency in rats produced plaques and abnormal vascularization associated with endothelial degeneration in the arteries. The researchers concluded that the primary nutritional role of selenium may be in assisting the growth and maintenance of the vascular membranes. Thus, there is strong suggestion that selenium prevents atherosclerotic plaques.

Selenium Is Vital to Heart Function

Coenzyme Q (an essential in certain enzymatic reactions) is indispensable to heart function. Not surprisingly, all heart-disease patients tested for Coenzyme Q revealed a deficiency detected in biopsy samples. Animal studies have further shown that a deficiency in Coenzyme Q lessens heart vitality and produces cardiac degenerative lesions. Because selenium appears to be the most important nutrient in the control of Coenzyme Q levels, adequate selenium is essential to produce the necessary Coenzyme Q required for a healthy heart.

Selenium Food Supplements Are Available

A drug which consists of vitamin E and selenium, Telsem (manufactured by Chromalloy), has been given a two-year clinical trial in Mexico. This combination was reported by the *Wall Street Journal* on March 13, 1973, to have produced 92 percent beneficial responses in patients with recurring attacks of angina pectoris—with or without myocardial infarct. These responses involved reduction or elimination of angina attacks, improved electrocardiograms, and increased vigor and work capacity. There was no evidence of adverse side effects. Although this drug is not available in the U.S. at this time, other vitamin E–selenium food supplements are.

The recent availability of selenium as a food supplement has been the most exciting news to me, for it is fruitless to research the protective capabilities of selenium and vitamin E against heart disease, cancer, and premature aging if the public cannot subsequently benefit. When I wrote *Supernutrition* (Dial, 1975; Pocket Books, 1976) and reported on my research with the combination of selenium and vitamin E, the only product commercially available was a veterinary

Table 11.1

A Comparison of Selenium with Vitamins C and E

	Natural Anti-oxidant	Deficient in Typical U.S. Diet	Linked, in a beneficial sense, with major health problems.
VITAMIN C	YES	YES[1]	Helps prevent common cold, high cholesterol levels, low resistance to disease, and detoxifies pollutants.
VITAMIN E	YES	YES[2]	Helps prevent heart attack, stroke, vascular diseases.
SELENIUM	YES	YES[3]	Helps prevent cancer, heart attack, infection, arthritis, and detoxifies pollutants.

(1) Twenty-seven per cent of U.S. diets supply less than recommended amounts. *U.S. Dept. of Agriculture Nationwide Study,* 1965.

(2) Typical U.S. diet supplies only 36% of USRDA. *Am. Journ. Clin. Nutr.,* July, 1965.

(3) Typical U.S. diet contains less than 0.1 part per million. *Lancet,* August, 1968. A level of 0.1 ppm prevents deficiency symptoms in animals.

Chart prepared by Dr. Herb Boynton, LaJolla, California.

drug, Seletoc, (containing 68 IU vitamin E and 1,000 micro grams selenium) used since 1962 to treat arthritis in dogs and to combat a disease with a dominant pathology of heart-muscle degeneration in lambs and calves. But today in health-food stores, you can buy Sel-E-Chrome (manufactured by Alacer, Buena Park, California), selenium (made by Solgar, Lynbrook, N.Y., American Dietaids and others), vitamin E plus selenium (produced by Schiff Bio-Food, Moonachie, N.J.), and selenium-enriched yeast (from Nutrition 21, La Jolla, California). A comparison of the properties and availability in the standard American diet of selenium and vitamins C and E is given in Table 11.1.

In areas containing adequate selenium in the soil, typical

selenium intake in the daily diet averages from 20 to 100 micrograms. As a food supplement, another 50 to 150 micrograms daily can safely be taken. The maximum daily intake of selenium is about 1,100 micrograms (M.L. Scott, Symposium on Selenium, University of Notre Dame, 1976).

The ingestion of above 2,000 micrograms (2 milligrams) in the total diet is toxic in the long term. Therefore, do not exceed the dosage indicated on the supplement's label unless advised to do so by a physician.

The Natural Sources of Selenium

The refining and cooking of food by commercial processers causes serious losses of selenium. Typically, each process destroys one-half of the selenium. Good natural sources of selenium include garlic, onion, asparagus, mushrooms, wheat, corn, eggs, brewer's yeast, tuna, liver, shrimp, kidney, and the meat of all fowl and grazing animals. Of course, the foods vary in selenium content with the soil or feed in which they grow. (TV dinners and canned fruits and vegetables are usually very low in this trace element.)

In fact, very few of us get adequate amounts of selenium, although research strongly indicates that selenium deficiency increases the probability of cancer and heart disease. To prevent heart-disease deaths, we must take adequate amounts of the major antioxidant nutrients—vitamin E, selenium, and vitamin C. Before we examine vitamin C, however, let's look at another important nutrient—pangamate (vitamin B_{15}).

12

Pangamate (Vitamin B₁₅)– The Little-Known Nutrient

Pangamate is an important, but virtually unknown, nutrient that has been shown to prevent and cure heart disease. It also postpones the signs of aging, reduces fatigue, and improves your sense of well-being.

The curative and protective functions of pangamate sound very much like those of vitamin E, although pangamate is not an antioxidant. But while pangamate and vitamin E have similar and complementary effects, their pathways of action are very different.

Pangamate improves the available oxygen content of the blood, enhances the circulatory blood volume, lowers arterial pressure, normalizes the heart's balance of potassium and sodium, suppresses heart pains in coronary disease, and accelerates heart and vascular system repair (by stimulating protein metabolism in the heart).

Pangamate increases the efficiency of tissue respiration; thus less oxygen is required by the body. (F.N. Marshal et al., *Federation Proceedings,* 1961; M. Idzumia, *Vitamins* [Japan], 1959) Additionally, pangamate methylates pollutants in the blood that compete with the body cells for the oxygen that is available in the bloodstream. If the pollutants are methylated they consume less oxygen; thus the circulating blood has more available oxygen. These two factors combine to have a very beneficial effect on the oxygen needs of the body (Dr. A. A. Apanasenko, Faculty Therapy

Dept., Medical Institute, Blagoveshchensk-on-Amur, USSR, *Cor Vasa,* 1973).

My interest in pangamate was first aroused by reading reports of Russian experiments in which it had been successfully used to reduce the effects of premature aging. Because pangamate increases the amount of oxygen available in the blood (by stimulating tissue respiration and reducing the oxygen consumption of pollutants), it reduces the detrimental effect of a diminished blood supply due to narrowed arteries. Thus, diseases once associated with aging, such as angina (resulting from insufficient oxygen to the heart) and senility (resulting from insufficient oxygen to the brain) are relieved.

My interest in pangamate was further heightened by impressive results obtained while working with veteran professional athletes. Not only does pangamate supply more "available" oxygen to muscles for work, it reduces fatigue and builds muscles. It seems to be tailor-made for veteran pros "ground down" by years of championship-caliber competition.

However, the most important use of pangamate is not in preventing premature aging or in helping athletes, but in curing heart disease.

Early Dramatic Results

The effect of pangamate on heart-disease patients was studied in the mid-1960s by Soviet physician Dr. Yakov Shpirt (of the Moscow Clinical Hospital No. 60). The impressive results of several of his studies were published in 1964 and 1965, and confirmed by other Soviet researchers and the Soviet Scientific Advisory Committee of the Ministry of Health in 1968.

The first large-scale study conducted by Dr. Shpirt and his colleagues Drs. O. L. Bobrova and E. A. Fizdel involved patients who had arteriosclerosis (hardening of the arteries due to calcification of cholesterol deposits). This group included those suffering from angina pectoris (pain and pressure about the heart), essential hypertension (high blood pressure), obliterative atherosclerosis (complete blockage of a blood vessel) to the legs and feet, and tachycardia (abnormal rapidity of heart action resulting in insufficient blood through-put).

The research program used pangamate to treat 118 cases of coronary sclerosis (hardening of the arteries) with its complications of hypertension and diabetes. Of the 118 patients, 104 experienced substantial improvement. Fifty-five patients had definite Improvements in electrocardiogram, blood chemistry, heart-pain relief, disappearance of dyspnea (labored breathing), and general well-being. An additional forty-nine patients experienced the subjective benefits of pain relief, dyspnea disappearance, and improvement of their general condition, but showed little or no objective progress in electrocardiogram and blood chemistry during the 10 to 20 days of the treatment. Those patients in the earlier stages of heart disease responded to pangamate alone, while those having a history of heart attacks also required vitamins A and E and other medications to obtain improvement.

Those still concerned about cholesterol may be interested that Dr. Shpirt reported that pangamate was given to 42 heart patients with an average cholesterol value of 211 milligrams of cholesterol per 100 milliliters of blood. After 20 days of taking 90 milligrams of pangamate daily, the average cholesterol level dropped to 175, and after 30 days (10 days after pangamate supplementation was terminated) the improved metabolism dropped the average cholesterol level to 168.

Heart Disease Is Relieved by Pangamate

In other experiments, pangamate has relieved several types of heart disease from atherosclerosis and angina pectoris to tachycardia and myocardial infarction by increasing the volume of available oxygen to compensate for poor circulation.

A myocardial infarction is an area of heart muscle that has

died because of stoppage of blood resulting from coronary thrombosis (a blood clot in a coronary artery). If the infarct is minor, the dead tissue can be replaced by a patch of scar tissue and the heart can become normal again. Rest is required so as not to exert the heart and cause it to rupture through the weak dead tissue before it is replaced by scar tissue. And blood-thinning drugs can be given to lessen the burden on the heart while it heals.

The effect of pangamate on 42 patients with myocardial infarctions was studied in 1973 by Dr. A. A. Apanasenko. Examinations were performed before and at the conclusion of the treatment, using electrocardiography, polycardiography, and measurements of arterial pressure and circulation rate. Pangamate was administered in daily doses of 150 milligrams for 20 to 30 consecutive days. In addition, sixteen patients with severe heart disease received single injections of strophanthin (a drug that strengthens heart action). Electrocardiograph and other indicators were examined both before and 30 minutes after the intravenous injection of strophanthin.

It was found that pangamate helped by itself but was not as good as strophanthin by itself, and results were better when both were given. The pangamate treatment led to a strengthening of heart contractions, as documented by clinical findings showing an improvement in both coronary and general blood circulation, and as indicated by polycardiographic examination exhibiting changes in the phase structure of heart contractions. Pangamate also prevented the side effects of strophanthin. The findings justify the recommendation that pangamate be used for treating patients with coronary disease; if marked heart failure is present, concurrent use of cardiotonic glucosides (drugs) is indicated (*Cor Vasa,* 1973).

Pangamate Speeds Healing of the Heart

In 1969 Drs. G. P. Chernyshev, V. I. Kuz'min, and S. A. Polilei published a report showing that pangamate had a pronounced effect on the heart's healing process. The researchers surgically caused an infarct in experimental dogs by tying off a coronary artery. They had divided the dogs into six groups; one group serving as a control received no treatment; other groups received pangamate, one of two drugs (strophanthin or gomphotin), or one of the drugs plus pangamate.

In dogs receiving pangamate, "considerably less regions were subject to the infarct effect and the dystrophic process in the muscular fibers adjacent to the infarct zone were very much less pronounced. Reparative processes in the myocardium [heart muscle] were characterized by pronounced activity, and the scar formed in place of the infarct had a loose distribution of fibers and an abundance of cellular elements and vessels." (Nauch. Tr., Omsk Medical Institute, 1969.)

In a later report that year, the researchers explained that with the combination of one drug and pangamate, blood pressure in the experimental dogs returned to normal within 10 to 15 days after the induced infarct, whereas in those receiving the drugs alone 3 weeks were required to return blood pressure to normal. Additionally, the animals receiving the drug plus pangamate had their blood-flow velocity normalized by the third day, whereas in those receiving only the drug, that required 10 days. Other chemical signs of cure, such as levels of the enzyme SGOT were faster in the pangamate-treated animals.

Pangamate Normalizes Fat Metabolism

In 1974, Dr. N. Nankov (of the Medical Clinic at the Institute of Veterinary Medicine at Sofia, Bulgaria) revealed that minks fed a diet that normally produces fatty livers were protected by supplements of pangamate. With pangamate, fat transport from liver cells increased, fat metabolism in fat depots increased, and total metabolism increased through the cholesterol secretion by the liver *(Monatsh. Veterinaermed.).*

Previously, Dr. V. I. Yakubovskaya of Karaganda, USSR, reported (in 1972) that an experiment with laboratory rats showed that "the effects of pangamate were correlated to its dose, with only a 200 mg [daily] dose markedly inhibiting fatty degeneration of the liver, decreasing its fat content by 50%. At that time it normalized all other indexes of fat metabolism."

Pangamate Improves Circulation

Improved blood circulation was noted by Russian researcher Dr. K. Yakupova after administering a daily dose of 100 milligrams of pangamate rectally to human volunteers. The enhanced blood circulation in the brain was measured rheoencephalographically. The increased circulation to the vital organs was gained by diminishing the supply to the peripheral muscles. This was probably due to hormonal action, most likely epinephrine, from adrenal or hypophysis stimulation (*Prob. Psikhoneurol.,* 1969).

Sources of Pangamate

Pangamate is found only in natural whole foods, which most people avoid or can't get anymore. This important nutrient, along with several others, has been stripped from most foods by either processing or by discarding the vitamin-rich seeds. Furthermore, it has been missing from most vitamin supplements in North America.

In nature, pangamate is found along with other members of the vitamin B complex. In the late 1940s, it was isolated from apricot pits and identified as the chemical substance pangamic acid by Dr. Ernst T. Krebs, Sr., and colleagues. Later, they isolated the substance from rice, brewer's yeast, horse liver, and steer blood. Dr. Krebs designated the substance vitamin B_{15} because it was the fifteenth member of the vitamin B complex to be identified.

Calcium pangamate, an improved form, was introduced

Table 12.1

Some Natural Sources of Pangamate
(milligrams per 100 grams or 3.5 ounces
of fresh, untreated food)

Rice Bran	200
Corn Grits	150
Oat Grits	106
Wheat Germ	70
Wheat Bran	31
Barley Grits	12
Wheat Flour	10

in 1964 by biochemists at the Biochemical Institute of the
USSR Academy of Sciences. According to a 1966 issue of
the Russian publication *Culture and Life,* calcium pangamate met with dramatic initial success in the treatment of
intermittent claudication (restless legs and pain in the legs)
and arteriosclerosis of the legs. Soon medical researchers
in France, Venezuela, Yugoslavia, Rumania, and Austria
were reporting similar successes with calcium pangamate.

How Pangamate Works

It is clear that the function of pangamate is to increase the
available supply of oxygen in the blood. The additional oxygen benefits people with heart disease who have less blood
getting through narrowed arteries, it helps aging athletes,
it overcomes gangrene, and it maintains cellular health to
prevent premature aging.

By definition, a vitamin is an essential ingredient required
in the diet to prevent disease, but to date convincing evidence that vitamin B_{15} is essential to humans is lacking.
Thus, vitamin B_{15} is not presently recognized by the FDA as
a vitamin. Some researchers refer to it as a provitamin (a
substance converted into a vitamin by the body) or a cofactor (a substance aiding the body in the use of other nutri-

ents, but not, in itself, essential in the diet). And most researchers have dropped the looser term "vitamin B₁₅" and use the term pangamic acid or pangamate (a salt of pangamic acid). This is similar to the biochemists' preference for "tocopherol" for vitamin E and "ascorbic acid" for vitamin C.

Effective Dosage Levels

Much research remains to be done on the physiological action of pangamate. There is general agreement on the most effective dosage, but debate as to what happens when that optimum dosage is exceeded. Pangamate is a nontoxic water-soluble member of the B-complex family, and you would expect excess pangamate to be harmless and merely excreted. This is what most researchers believe.

However, an experiment reported by Drs. E. A. Kutateladze and M. I. Dzhabua showed that there can be differences in the physiological action of large doses of pangamate on lipid (fat) metabolism (*Soobshch. Akad. Nauk Gruz.,* 1970).

Typically, therapeutic dosages call for 100 to 150 milligrams daily for three to four weeks, followed by a maintenance dosage of 50 milligrams daily as a supplement to the diet. Drs. Kutateladze and Dzhabua confirmed this optimum rate with a detailed study of cholesterol, phospholipids, and lipoproteins in the blood, liver, heart, and kidneys of adult rats fed a complete and balanced diet in addition to the pangamate supplement. The surprising finding, which as yet remains unexplained, is that at ten times that level of supplementation, the beneficial changes were less. Their experiment indicates that 140 milligrams of pangamate for a 154-pound person results in much more marked, favorable, and prolonged changes in lipid metabolism than 1,400 milligrams.

The scientific literature reports that 100 milligrams of calcium pangamate taken orally every day was found to be nontoxic according to standard clinical tests. **Some pa-**

tients taking large doses (exceeding 500 mg/day) have experienced a mild flushing of the skin, similar to the reaction to niacin; others have noted a temporary drowsiness when first beginning pangamate therapy. Because each person responds differently to nutrients or drugs, care should be taken when beginning any supplement to see if you tolerate it or are allergic to it.

Pangamate is available from several manufacturers, Including Aangmik (Food Science Laboratories Inc. and Da Vinci Inc., S. Burlington, Vt.), and Belvedere Laboratories (Hayward, Cal.).

If you are free of heart disease, you should consider adding 50 milligrams of calcium pangamate daily to your diet, especially if you are over forty years of age. If you have heart disease, you should consider taking a daily therapeutic dose of 150 milligrams for a month, followed by a maintenance dose of 50 milligrams daily. Pangamate is part of the Supernutrition Plan outlined in the final chapter.

13
Other B Vitamins Are Important Too!

Most foods containing one B vitamin contain a family of water-soluble vitamins called the B-complex. It's important to have generous amounts of all of the B-complex vitamins but the major members, with respect to heart disease, will be discussed here. Liver, yeast, and whole grains are excellent sources of the B-complex.

Pyridoxine (B$_6$)

Vitamin B$_6$ (pyridoxine) is needed to properly metabolize the fats and sugars in our diet, and to produce lecthin needed for normal lipid balance. (It can be found in B-complex tablets.)

Vitamin B$_3$

Niacin, niacinamide, and nicotinic acid all have vitamin B$_3$ activity. Generally they are interchangeable, but niacin and nicotinic acid are preferred for lowering cholesterol. For those interested in cholesterol levels, niacin (vitamin B$_3$) has been shown to lower blood levels of cholesterol slightly. But more importantly, it also increased the chances for survival from heart disease and improves circulation.

The Veterans Administration (VA) of the United States has for several years been investigating nicotinic-acid therapy in the secondary prevention of coronary attacks. The VA study after four years shows a survival rate of 84 percent for those heart patients receiving niacin therapy as compared to a 75 percent survival rate for the controls. The decrease in blood cholesterol after a year of treatment with niacin ranges from 15 to 25 percent. The B-complex vitamins inositol and para-amino-benzoic acid have similar effects on lipid balance.

The administration of large amounts of niacin differs from that of vitamins C and E in that there are side effects. These side effects, which are reversible after the initial heavy dosages are reduced or disappear after several weeks of therapy, include cutaneous flushing (reddening of the skin), remission of rheumatism and arthritis, hyperglycemia, and impaired glucose tolerance. These effects indicate that niacin stimulates the release of the hormone ACTH. On the other hand, niacinamide does not produce the side effects. (Niacin or niacinamide can also be found in B-complex tablets.)

Orotic Acid (B_{13})

Orotic acid (vitamin B_{13}) promotes recovery from heart attacks, according to studies at the University of New South Wales, Australia (*Chemical and Engineer News,* 1974). Orotic acid speeds enlargement of surviving muscle cells. Thus, the heart adjusts better to the extra work forced upon the undamaged portion of the heart after an infarct, valve damage, or high blood pressure. Animals given therapeutic amounts at the acute stage following heart damage have shown immediate improvement in heart function and quicker recovery. An especially effective form of orotic acid is its magnesium salt, magnesium orotate.

Vitamin B_{13} is not widely available, except in low 1–5 milligram dosages. It is generally not in B-complex tablets. Be sure to eat liver, yeast, and whole grains to obtain all of the B-complex. The lower dosages will suffice for the healthy person, but heart patients may wish to ask their doctors about prescriptions of magnesium orotate.

The B-complex vitamins play an important role in heart health. The Supernutrition Program presented in Chapter 32 will aid you in determining the optimum amount of the B-complex vitamins for you. As a general guide, a healthy person should take a B-complex tablet containing at least 25–50 milligrams of each of the B vitamins (the RDAs are generally 2–20 milligrams). A person with heart trouble should consider taking amounts of 50 to 100 milligrams. The B-complex vitamins should be taken in divided doses (2–4 times daily) because they are water-soluble and are retained in the body for only short periods.

14
Vitamin C for Healthy Arteries

Vitamin C is critical in the prevention of heart disease, yet there is a significant deficiency of vitamin C in the American diet. This important nutrient combats stress, maximizes vitamin E activity, and reverses cholesterol buildup in plaques.

Individuals prone to heart attack usually have extremely low serum vitamin C levels. Within six to twelve hours after heart attacks, blood vitamin C levels drop to values typical of persons with scurvy. This information was revealed in 1972 by Dr. R. Hume (of Southern General Hospital, Glasgow, Scotland) in the *British Heart Journal;* he concluded that the vitamin C lost to the bloodstream has been absorbed by the heart to assist in healing the damage.

Like those prone to heart attack, smokers have lower vitamin C levels than the rest of the population; older peoples' diets tend to be more deficient in vitamin C than those of younger people; men often have lower serum levels of vitamin C than women on identical diets; and people under stress experience lower vitamin C levels than those not under stress. For years, Soviet scientists have published articles on the relationship of atherosclerosis and vitamin C; now they routinely prescribe vitamin C when the disease appears.

Vitamin C and the Stress Cycle

Stress (which is different from hard work or competitive stimuli) is a valid heart-disease factor. Under stress conditions (frustration, insecurity, aimlessness, mental tension, physical injury, or surgery) the adrenal glands secrete epinephrine (adrenalin), in the process consuming vitamin C, which is stored in the adrenal glands. In fact, the body's vitamin C supply can be exhausted in only a few seconds of stress. If the stress continues, then the demands of the adrenal glands take priority over those of other tissues, utilizing the vitamin C needed elsewhere in the body and, in consequence, impairing the health of other tissues. When the vitamin C supply is exhausted, the adrenal gland fails to perform adequately in response to stress by raising blood pressure, blood supply, etc., for defense. Since we cannot avoid all stress, we should be sure to maintain a high level of vitamin C in the blood. The proper amount for you can be determined with the Supernutrition Program (see p. 301).

Vitamin C Maximizes Vitamin E Activity

Vitamin C has a synergistic effect on the antioxidant action of vitamin E. This simply means that vitamins C and E working together have greater total effect than the sum of their individual effects. Consequently, vitamin C is instrumental in preventing the cellular membrane damage that causes the proliferation of the arterial smooth muscle cells and eventually plaque formation.

Vitamin C Is Essential for Healthy Arteries

Vitamin C is needed for artery health, and a deficiency makes the arterial walls abnormally permeable. In turn, this results in the loss of the natural protecting substances normally in the artery lining, thus allowing harmful mutagens to enter through the walls. A vitamin C deficiency has an adverse effect on the composition of the intercellular matrix substance of tissue (ground substance) and impairs metabolism in the arterial wall. Vitamin C has long been known to be necessary in maintaining capillary health, and a deficiency results in loss of blood through capillary breakage.

Low Vitamin C Levels Are Linked to Higher Mortality Rates

Early nutritional experiments on humans showed that a vitamin C deficiency could trigger heart attacks in healthy volunteers aged 20 to 30 years (Sir Hans Krebs, *Journal of Biochemistry,* 1946; Drs. C. Krumdieck and C. E. Butterworth, *American Journal of Clinical Nutrition,* 1974). According to a large statistical survey by E. G. Knox, the more vitamin C in the diet, the fewer heart attacks and strokes. Statistical data comparing mortality ratios in various parts of Great Britain with standardized ratios of mortality due to ischemic heart disease and cerebrovascular disease show significantly higher mortality in regions of low vitamin C intake than in regions having higher vitamin C intake (*Lancet,* 1973).

Vitamin C Removes Plaque and Cholesterol from Arteries

Vitamin C has been shown to reverse plaque formation. Although vitamin C has been demonstrated to dissolve cholesterol and calcium in test tubes, few scientists have believed that the same process could occur in the body. Yet several studies have shown that vitamin C does remove the cholesterol and calcium part of the plaque, leaving mostly monoclonal cells and collagen behind. During a study among 20 patients with atherosclerosis, 6 of the 10 patients given vitamin C supplements experienced partial regressions of their plaques, while none of the 10 patients not receiving vitamin C improved (C. Krumdieck and C. E. Butterworth, *American Journal of Clinical Nutrition,* 1974).

Animal experiments have also shown that vitamin C clears plaque material from arterial walls. The cholesterol content of aortas in experimental rats decreases after vitamin C administration, according to researchers B. Nambisan and P. A. Kurup (*Atherosclerosis,* 1974). In 1971, Dr. Ralph Mumma (a Pennsylvania State University biologist) reported that vitamin C flushed cholesterol from the inner arterial walls of experimental rats.

The removal of calcium and cholesterol (and other plaque material) reduces the chance of heart attacks in two ways. First, as plaque is removed, the artery obstructs the blood flow less. The difference of a small amount of plaque can be very significant. The blood flowing through the artery varies with the fourth power of the diameter. Thus, when a plaque half-fills an artery, the blood flow is only one-sixteenth of what it was. Less blood means heart pain (angina). Second, plaque material enhances clot formation because of reduced flow and the collagen (protein fiber) in the plaque. Clots cause heart attacks.

For those concerned about blood cholesterol levels, vitamin C is of special interest, for it has been shown to regulate in part the amount of cholesterol circulating in the blood. In persons with a deficiency of vitamin C, the body's ability to convert cholesterol to bile is impaired; instead of being properly used, the cholesterol in these individuals accumulates in the bloodstream. Vitamin C tends to counteract the effect, and to normalize the blood cholesterol level.

Vitamin C Deficiency Is Linked to Plaque Formation

Perhaps the greatest research in this area has been done by Dr. Emil Ginter (Director of the Biochemical Department of the Research Institute of Human Nutrition in Bratislava, Czechoslovakia). In 1959, Dr. Ginter and his associates began a detailed study of the metabolic consequences of chronic vitamin C deficiency. Their research earned them worldwide recognition, yet the American medical profession has not followed up their studies.

Dr. Ginter set out to see if there was a relationship between vitamin C deficiency and atherosclerosis. He chose the guinea pig for his experimental model because, like man (and unlike most other animals), the guinea pig does not make its own vitamin C. Ginter noted that others had conducted similar studies, but the results could not be relied on (although the researchers attested to the value of vitamin C) because the experimental animals had been made completely deficient in vitamin C and consequently developed scurvy, which produced drastic changes in the animals' biochemistry. Ginter made his animals only slightly deficient so as to avoid scurvy.

In 1965, Dr. Ginter conducted an experiment with two groups, each composed of 30 guinea pigs on low-fat diets. The control group was fed a diet containing 5 milligrams of vitamin C, while the experimental group was deprived of vitamin C for two weeks, then fed one-tenth the vitamin C given the control group. One year after the experiment had begun, the amount of cholesterol in the arterial plaques averaged 30 percent higher in the vitamin-C–deficient group.

A second experiment was designed to see what effect vitamin C would have on a high-cholesterol diet. Again two groups of guniea pigs were used, but the amounts of vitamin C were increased to handle the extra dietary fat. The control group received 50 milligrams of vitamin C while the experimental group received 5 milligrams. After one year, an average of 550 milligrams of plaque had accumulated in the aortic wall of the vitamin-C–deficient group as opposed to an average of only 400 milligrams in the vitamin-C–enriched group. This suggests that vitamin C deficiency enhanced the formation of cholesterol in the proliferating monoclonal smooth muscle cells.

An Important Realization

Dr. Constance R. Leslie (formerly Spittle—a pathologist at Pinderfields General Hospital in Wakefield, Yorkshire, England) suggested in a 1971 letter to the editor of the *Hospital Tribune* that "Humans taking large doses of vitamin C will not necessarily get a fall in serum cholesterol—indeed, they may get the reverse, because they are mobilizing their arterial cholesterol. The actual serum level is not relevant when they are taking the vitamin, since the cholesterol is being channeled in the right direction—away from the arteries."

Dr. Leslie first realized the possible "washing out" of cholesterol from artery walls when she observed that her own blood cholesterol would increase after taking vitamin C, regardless of her fat or cholesterol intake. She recruited a group of volunteers for a follow-up experiment that lasted 12 weeks, and included 58 healthy volunteers and 25 patients with atherosclerosis.

During the first 6 weeks, none of the volunteers received a vitamin C supplement to their normal diets, but during the second 6-week period, they all took 1 gram of vitamin C daily. Most healthy volunteers under 25 years of age showed decreases in their blood cholesterol levels, with an average decrease of 8 percent. Most of the atherosclerotic volunteers experienced a rise in serum cholesterol, averaging nearly 10 percent (most likely as arterial cholesterol was dissolved and entered the bloodstream). Similarly, some of the expected rise in blood cholesterol level was found in the healthy volunteers over 45 years of age. Healthy volunteers between 25 and 45 showed mixed results, presumably because in some, cholesterol was being washed out of their arteries, while in others (who had nearly "clean" arteries to begin with), blood cholesterol levels were being lowered. Dr. Leslie's report was published in *Lancet* in 1971.

An earlier Scottish study among 20 atherosclerotic patients had produced similar findings. Within one month after taking 500 milligrams of vitamin C thrice daily, blood cholesterol levels dropped an average of 30 percent

(B. McConnell and B. Sokoloff, *Proceedings of the Sixth International Congress of Nutrition,* Edinburgh, 1963).

A Therapeutic Combination

Dr. Kurt Oster (Chief of Cardiology Emeritus, Park City Hospital in Connecticut) has had excellent results curing atherosclerosis using vitamin C with folic acid (a B-complex vitamin). In the October 1976 issue of *American Laboratory,* Dr. Oster reported, "Sixty patients are at present under study with the combination of folic acid and ascorbic acid. Daily doses of 80 mg of folic acid produced remarkable clinical effects, especially measurable and observable in peripheral arteriosclerosis of diabetic patients."

Dr. Oster has described "folic acid as the 'penicillin equivalent' for the treatment of amenable atherosclerotic clinical manifestations." As he reported, "The combination has excellent therapeutic effects without damage to the patient— [it is] the ideal drug."

Vitamin C Reduces Clot Formation

Dr. Leslie has also shown that vitamin C administration reduces the tendency to form lethal blood clots (both arterial and venous) in those particularly susceptible (*Lancet,* 1973). In one experiment, clot-prone patients were divided into two groups. Those not receiving vitamin C supplements had 60 percent clot incidence while those receiving vitamin C had only 33 percent clot incidence.

The Vitamin C Scare Is Groundless

From time to time the medical establishment issues scare reports warning of the risk of taking more than the RDA of vitamin C. One report by Dr. Victor Herbert of Columbia University warned that large doses of vitamin C would destroy the body's supply of vitamin B_{12} and cause serious nerve damage (*Journal of the American Medical Association,* 1974). The warning stemmed from a crude test-tube experiment unrelated to body conditions, and later Dr. Jerome J. DeCosse (of the Medical College of Wisconsin's Department of Surgery and Pathology) proved this warning to have been a false scare. Dr. DeCrosse found none of his patients who had received large amounts of vitamin C to be deficient in vitamin B_{12}, even though they were not taking vitamin B_{12} supplements.

Additionally, Dr. Mehr Afronz and his colleagues (of the St. Louis University Group Hospitals) reported in the *Journal of the American Medical Association* in 1975 that they have been giving more than 4,000 milligrams of vitamin C daily to all spinal-cord-injury patients under their care, with no adverse effect on vitamin B_{12} levels. They measured vitamin B_{12} levels of their long-term patients, all of whom had been taking 4,000 milligrams of vitamin C for 11 months or more, and found not one patient deficient in vitamin B_{12}.

Occasionally the claim is made that increased vitamin C intake increases the risk of kidney stones, but Drs. Charles E. Butterworth and Carlos Krundieck (of the School of Medicine of the University of Alabama in Birmingham) have reported that even taking 3,000 milligrams of vitamin C a day produces no increase in oxalates, the main material of kidney stones, in urine (*American Journal of Clinical Nutrition,* 1974).

Dr. Abram Hoffer reports that in 20 years of experience of prescribing huge doses of vitamin C he has not seen any oxalate urinary stones in his patients.

Dr. Linus Pauling explained the harmlessness of vitamin C before the Senate Subcommittee on Health, chaired by Senator Edward Kennedy, in 1975, as follows:

"Vitamin C has been described as one of the least toxic substances known. People have ingested 125 grams (over a quarter of a pound) at one time without harm, and an equal amount has been injected intravenously into a human being without harm. It is unlikely that ingestion in the amounts of two grams to twenty grams per day, the amounts [daily] synthesized by animals, over long periods of time would lead to harm. It has been suggested that a high intake of vitamin C continued for a long time might lead to the formation of kidney stones, but in fact not a single case has been reported in the medical literature. . . . A careful study showed that the amount of oxalate was increased very little by an intake of four grams of vitamin C per day, and is only doubled for an intake of ten grams per day, for normal subjects."

Dr. W. J. McCormick published his finding that patients with urinary stones had, on the average, a *low* level of vitamin C in the blood (*The Medical Record*, 1946).

Further information on vitamin C studies can be found in Irwin Stone's book, *The Healing Factor: Vitamin C Against Disease* (Grosset and Dunlap, 1972). The disadvantages of increased vitamin C intake appear to be unverifiable, but the advantages have proved to be striking.

15

Calcium, Magnesium, and Potassium— Essential Macro-Minerals

Like the trace (micro-)mineral selenium, the macro-minerals calcium, magnesium, and potassium are essential for heart health. The largest source of minerals is our diet, but a significant portion comes from our drinking water and the water in which we cook our food.

Calcium Deficiency Correlates Highly with Heart Disease

A strong correlation between calcium deficiency and heart disease was found by Dr. E. G. Knox (of the Health Services Research Center of the University of Birmingham in England). Of the nutrients studied, calcium deficiency produced the leading association with heart disease, while vitamin C deficiency was the predominant factor in causes of death from all diseases (*Lancet,* 1973).

Calcium is a macro-mineral, which means that more than mere traces are needed in the daily diet for optimum health. The 1974 RDA for adults suggests 800 milligrams of calcium, but several researchers feel that at least 1,200 milligrams (approximately the amount in a quart of milk) are required (H. Spencer, *Federation Proceedings,* March 1974; L. Lutwak, "Osteoporosis," *Disease-a-Month,* 1963).

A secondary benefit of calcium is that it decreases lead

absorption, thus offering protection against lead poisoning, which emanates from automobile exhaust and which prevents red blood cells from being formed.

Vitamin D is required for proper calcium utilization, as are magnesium, vitamin C, fats, and other nutrients. This is why total nutrition is important, and illustrates how any deficiency can eventually lead to heart disease.

I prefer cow's milk as a calcium source. The Supernutrition Score will help individuals find what is best for them. (For me—I drink at least half a gallon of milk a day and take daily calcium supplements.) For supplements, I prefer the chelated calcium (that which is bound to such organic compounds as amino acids) or an organic salt such as calcium lactate or calcium gluconate, rather than the relatively inefficient bone meal, dolomite, or dicalcium phosphate. (Of course, any calcium is better than no calcium at all.)

There is evidence that phosphorus carries away calcium with it as the phosphorus is excreted. Since our diets are rich in phosphorus (which occurs in everything from cola to meat), calcium supplements without phosphorus are preferred.

Magnesium Is Essential for Heart Health

Magnesium is required for the heart muscle to relax so that it can contract again, and to prevent calcification in the heart valves. Magnesium produces peripheral vasodilation (increased circulation to the less vital blood vessels such as those in arms and legs) and lowered blood pressure. When calcium intake is high, the magnesium intake should also be high to prevent a magnesium deficiency, since the two minerals compete for absorption.

Magnesium is removed from grains in the refining process and is not replenished by "enrichment." Stress causes the body to use up its magnesium. And if you live in a soft-water area, you may not be getting enough magnesium to start with.

The effect of soft water on the magnesium levels of the

body has been reported in the scientific literature. In 1967, Drs. T. Crawford and M. D. Crawford reported that the coronary arteries of those living in soft-water areas contained less calcium and magnesium. They determined this by comparing arteries from those killed in accidents in both soft- and hard-water areas in England (*Lancet,* 1967).

In 1973, Drs. B. Chipperfield and J. R. Chipperfield (of the University of Hull, in England) reported lower levels of magnesium in the hearts of those dying of sudden heart failure (*Lancet,* 1973).

In a Canadian study in 1975, Dr. T. W. Anderson and colleagues analyzed the mineral content in the hearts of those killed in accidents in hard- and soft-water areas. The only significant difference observed was in magnesium content. There was more magnesium in the hearts of those from hard-water areas. The levels of calcium, zinc, copper, chromium, lead, and cadium were essentially the same (*Canadian Medical Association Journal,* 1975).

A paper showing that magnesium orotate produced an excellent or at least a satisfactory normalization of blood-vessel elasticity in all of 64 atherosclerotic patients so treated has been published by Dr. Hans A. Nieper of Hanover, Germany (*Agressologie* [1974], 15, 1, 73–78.).

The RDA for magnesium is 350 milligrams for adult males, but there is debate as to whether this amount is optimal. If the blood analysis in your annual physical examination indicates a magnesium deficiency, you should add to your diet magnesium-rich foods such as wheat germ, kelp, brewer's yeast, sunflower seeds, sesame seeds, pumpkin seeds, nuts and nut butters, beans, and peas. If your magnesium deficiency is serious, your doctor should suggest a supplement in tablet form. The preferred form of magnesium supplement is magnesium orotate, because it provides the benefits of both magnesium and orotic acid (see Chapter 13) and because it is readily absorbed. Chelated magnesium and magnesium aspartate are acceptable when magnesium orotate is not available.

Potassium Deficiency Can Lead to Heart Failure

Because magnesium is involved in the retention of potassium in the cells, a deficiency of magnesium results in a deficiency of potassium, which may be even worse than magnesium deficiency in terms of resulting heart damage. Stress, alcohol, nicotine, caffeine, and an excess of salt all tend to reduce the body's stores of potassium. This deficiency produces an electrolyte imbalance directly responsible for arrhythmia (heartbeat irregularity), heart failure, and cell death, as well as death to the individual.

The Apollo 16 astronauts loaded up with potassium before takeoff and carried potassium-enriched foods (unspecified in reports) aboard their April 1972 flight, in order to prevent the irregular heart rhythms that affected the Apollo 15 crew.

Apollo 15 astronauts David Scott and James Irwin had both suffered from heart irregularities on their way back to earth. Potassium deficiencies caused by the extra heavy work performed by the crew plus the stress of weightlessness, which normally increases potassium excretion, had produced their irregular heartbeats.

Dr. Charles A. Berry, the astronauts' physician, first noted a few isolated premature heartbeats from James Irwin while he was working hard on the moon. Shortly before liftoff from the moon, Irwin produced a series of ten irregular beats. Later during the return flight, after working for three hours transferring moon rocks from the LEM to the command module, Irwin suffered another series of arrhythmias.

David Scott's arrhythmias didn't occur until just before the splashdown of Apollo 15. Scott had been taking aspirin for his shoulder pain, and aspirin accelerates potassium depletion.

After preflight loading of potassium and potassium-enriched foods, Apollo 16 astronauts Charles Duke, John Young, and Ken Mattingly survived the 12-day flight without arrhythmias.

Potassium deficiency can occur rather swiftly. In one

study, healthy volunteers on a highly refined diet developed potassium deficiencies and the accompanying muscular weakness and extreme fatigue in less than a week. Refined grains have been robbed of 75 percent of their potassium.

In cases of severe potassium deficiency, muscles (including the heart) can become paralyzed. Some people, as a result of heredity, have unusual demands for potassium. One experiment on a group of people with high-potassium needs produced paralysis within 24 hours when they were fed either salty foods, refined sweets, or diuretic drugs.

Diuretics are often given to people with high blood pressure to help prevent the complications leading to heart disease. Yet diuretics remove potassium along with the fluids, thus producing the possibility of heart disease unless potassium is replaced. Diuretics are also used in pills for weight reduction and the relief of menstrual distress, so if you are taking either kind of pill, be sure the foods you eat contain plenty of potassium. Dairy products, eggs, and meats are not overly rich in potassium, but seeds, parsley, bananas, bran, and potato skins are.

Since potassium is a macro-mineral, considerable quantities are required for optimum health. There is evidence that it is preferable to balance our sodium (salt) intake with an equal amount of potassium. If you add salt to your food, it may be prudent to use a half-and-half mixture of salt and potassium chloride (a salt substitute).

Potassium in tablet form is not often suggested and you certainly should not take potassium tablets unless your doctor prescribes them. People with kidney disease must be especially sure not to take potassium supplements without consulting their physician.

Prescription medicines are available, but many are enteric-coated tablets that don't dissolve until they reach the intestine, where they can irritate the intestines and cause complicated ulcers. Many nutritionists feel that potassium is preferably administered as a salt substitute on foods or dissolved in water (but without additional flavoring it does not make a very tasty beverage). However, health-food stores generally carry safe (non-enteric-coated) tablets of potassium gluconate, potassium aspartate, or potassium orotate.

Physicians should know that protection against heart disease appears possible by taking equal amounts of potassium aspartate and magnesium aspartate (or the orotates). Daily ingestion of 2 to 4 grams of a mixture of potassium and magnesium aspartates has been recommended for the angina that occurs after a myocardial infarction by Dr. Ilana A. Nieper and K. Blumberger (*Electrolytes and Cardiovascular Diseases*, Williams and Wilkins Co., Baltimore, 1965).

A deficiency of calcium, magnesium, or potassium can seriously affect the health of your heart. The best protection you can get is a balanced diet supplemented by a mineral tablet as indicated in the Supernutrition Program.

16

The Hazards of Soft Water

During the past 20 years, researchers around the world have observed that people living in hard-water areas (whose water is rich in calcium and magnesium) have a much lower heart-disease death rate than those living in soft-water areas. The harder the water, the lower the heart-disease death rate holds true across the United States, Japan, Finland, Sweden, Central Europe, the Netherlands, the United Kingdom, and Canada. The strongest association is with calcium, but an association also exists for magnesium.

One of the unfortunate properties of soft water is its usually higher content of sodium (table salt is sodium chloride), which can upset the potassium-sodium electrolyte balance. When this balance is disrupted, the heart cannot conduct the electrical stimulus that causes it to beat properly, and irregular heartbeat or heart failure results.

Soft Water Has Been Linked to Heart Disease

The first report of the link between soft water and heart disease was probably that of Japan's Dr. J. Kobayashi in 1957. Since 1957, many confirming reports have appeared, including those by Dr. Donald R. Peterson in Seattle, Dr. Gunnar Biorck of Stockholm, Dr. Margaret D. Crawford of England, and Dr. Henry A. Schroeder of Dartmouth Medical School in Hanover, New Hampshire.

In 1960, Dr. Schroeder compared a survey of water supplies in 1,315 American cities with the heart-disease death rates in those cities (*Journal of the American Medical Association,* 1960). The basis for the comparison was the

1950–51 U.S. Geological Survey of city water supplies, which covered 90 percent of the U.S. metropolitan population and 58 percent of the total U.S. population.

Dr. Schroeder's study showed that the 23 states having harder-than-average water supplies had lower-than-average heart-disease death rates. (The only two exceptions to this rule were Indiana and Illinois.) Of the remaining 25 states with softer-than-average water supplies, two-thirds had higher-than-average heart-disease death rates.

Apparently the higher the calcium content of the water, the better. For example, the average hardness of water supplied to South Carolinians was 18 parts per million calcium, compared with 237 parts per million for New Mexicans, and the heart-disease death rates among white males 45 to 64 years of age was far higher in South Carolina (1,107.5 per 100,000) than in New Mexico (563.4 per 100,000). There is, in fact, a much higher correlation between water hardness and low heart-disease mortality than between low dietary cholesterol and low heart-disease death rate. (See Chapter 16.)

In 1966, Dr. Schroeder updated his study, finding similar correlation between water hardness and lower heart-disease death rates (*Journal of the American Medical Association*). In 1968, Dr. Margaret Crawford and colleagues published similar results from a study of 61 English towns (*Lancet,* 1968).

Five years later, Dr. Crawford and her colleagues published a study of 289 men from 12 English cities, nearly alike except that six of the cities had hard-water supplies. Beyond a slight difference in lifestyle (the men in the soft-water group participated in slightly more exercise), the men were fairly well matched. The important finding was that the heart-disease death rate was 50 percent higher in the towns with the softest water (720 to 862 heart-disease deaths per 100,000 in the soft-water towns compared to 499 to 597 in the hard-water towns). In addition, the men in the soft-water towns had higher pulse rates, higher blood cholesterol levels, and higher blood pressures (*Engineering Digest,* 1973).

Two years earlier, Dr. Leland J. McCabe (Director of

Epidemiology and Biometrics of the Water Supplies Programs Division of the United States Environmental Protection Agency—EPA) had announced:

"Our research shows that among men, the hard-water death rate due to heart disease was 583 per 100,000 of the population and the death rate in soft-water areas was 643 per 100,000.

"For women, the hard-water death rate due to heart disease was 361 per 100,000 of the population and the death rate due to heart disease in soft-water areas was 446 per 100,000."

Current statistics from various authorities indicate that 70 percent of Americans drink soft water, and one estimate (unnamed in a brief filed against the EPA to act against soft water) is that 15 percent of the heart-disease deaths among those drinking soft water could be prevented by drinking hard water. This means, if the estimate is accurate, that about 10 percent of all heart disease in America could be prevented by switching to hard water.

Two cities in Florida which had earlier converted to soft water switched back to hard water and experienced a 48 percent reduction in heart disease (Dr. Paige, *Look* magazine).

As a rule, domestic and imported bottled waters are mineral waters that are untreated and thus are hard waters. However, some bottled waters are distilled waters which are free of all minerals and very soft. If you drink distilled water, be sure to get lots of calcium and magnesium in your diet.

I should point out that not all scientists are convinced that water "hardness" is a meaningful category, because different minerals can be present in two water supplies classified at the same level of hardness. Additionally, there are reversals in the link between soft water and heart disease. One example is the twin cities of Kansas City, Kansas (having hard water), and Kansas City, Missouri (having soft water). Here the heart-disease death rate is 36 percent lower in the soft-water (50 percent softer) city. However, the main difference may be the extra cadmium in the harder water. Cadmium, according to a study by Dr. Henry Schroeder, raises blood pressure (*The Poisons Around Us,* Indiana University Press, 1974). And high blood pressure causes heart-disease complications.

There is the possibility that another factor is involved in the beneficial effects of hard water besides the obvious high levels of calcium and magnesium, but no other factor has been adequately demonstrated. And there are reasons to believe that the protection from heart disease actually results from the calcium and magnesium. Calcium is used by the heart in the muscle contraction that produces the heartbeat, and magnesium repels the calcium to reverse the contraction to allow the heart to relax.

If soap lathers easily in your water, it's probably soft. Contact your local water department or the United States Geological Agency (or even the EPA) if you're interested in learning whether your local supply could be switched back to hard water. If such a switch is not possible, you should be especially sure your diet contains extra calcium and magnesium.

17

Zinc, Copper, and Chromium— Essential Trace Minerals

Several trace minerals, in addition to selenium, make important contributions to heart health. Chief among these are zinc, copper, and chromium.

Zinc and Copper

Many facts need to be uncovered before we can speak with certainty about zinc and copper, for test results and opinions continue to be conflicting. Two independent researchers have established what they feel are the ideal zinc-to-copper ratio. Dr. Leslie M. Klevay (of the USDA's Human Nutrition Laboratory in Grand Forks, N.D.) feels the ideal zinc-to-copper ratio is 6 to 1, because higher ratios increase blood cholesterol levels. Yet we know that blood cholesterol levels are really not that important in causing heart disease. The fact that 23 different minerals can raise the blood cholesterol tends to minimize the importance of the cholesterol rise caused by a zinc-to-copper ratio in excess of 6 to 1.

Dr. Carl Pfeiffer (of the Brain Bio Center in Princeton, N.J.) feels that the zinc-to-copper ratio should be as high as possible in order to remove excess copper from the body. He believes copper in excess of the 2–5-milligram-daily level is harmful because he has found that 50 percent of schizophrenics have excess copper in their bodies. Still, it is possible that the copper may accumulate in schizophrenics as a result of metabolic problems, rather than being the cause of their problems.

I agree with the premise that many of us are zinc-deficient and that 50 to 100 milligrams daily (the RDA is 15 mg) is often useful. The body selects what it needs when these amounts are available, and the ratio to zinc no longer is a factor. I think we should take in 1 to 5 milligrams daily of copper.

Zinc deficiency was indicated as a causative factor in atherosclerosis by Dr. W. Wacker in 1956 and reported in the *New England Journal of Medicine.* In 1971, Dr. Schroeder implicated zinc deficiency with hypertension. (His explanation appeared in *Clinical Chemistry.*)

Zinc's primary function in reducing high blood pressure results from the relief it offers from cadmium poisoning. Cadmium poisoning occurs as a result of water pollution and leaching from galvanized pipes. Cadmium appears in soft water and processed foods—especially cola drinks, instant coffees and teas, decaffeinated coffees, and food wrapped in plastic, tin, and aluminum cans. Cadmium is also present in cigarette smoke and air pollution—especially near new highways where tires are wearing (cadmium is used as a stabilizer for rubber). Zinc also promotes the healing of heart damage. Copper helps keep the arteries flexible.

Many researchers believe that if you consume high amounts of calcium and magnesium, you will induce a zinc deficiency, because the minerals compete for absorption. However, Dr. H. Spencer found that this was only a problem among persons eating vegetarian diets with high amounts of vegetable proteins, especially soybeans, containing large amounts of phytate (*Journal of Nutrition,* 1965). In a balanced diet containing animal protein, calcium does not interfere with zinc.

Whole grains and meats are good sources of zinc. Copper can be found in milk, fruits, and vegetables. **Only if the blood analysis in your annual physical exam indicates a** deficiency, and only then upon your doctor's advice, should you supply your body with supplemental amounts of zinc and copper in the form of low dosages of their chelates.

It is best to rely on nature, and provide your body with a diverse and balanced diet. Avoid taking large quantities of micro-nutrients, as little is known about possible toxicity or interrelationships. But avoid deficiencies as well. You should be sure the micro-nutrients are in your multivitamin and mineral formulation.

Essential Chromium Is Removed during the Refining of Flour and Sugar

It is difficult to induce atherosclerosis in experimental rats, but it can be done easily if they are made chromium-deficient (H. A. Schroeder, *The Trace Elements and Man,* Devin-Adair Co., Conn., 1973). Chromium is required for normal carbohydrate and fat metabolism. People in countries with high heart-disease death rates often eat a large amount of refined processed foods containing white sugar and white flour, from which the trace mineral chromium has been removed. Western man gets only about one-tenth of the chromium he needs for a balanced diet, and to make matters worse, 50 percent of the modern diet is processed food. Thus a negative chromium balance is a common occurrence.

Dr. Schroeder found chromium present in all young persons tested, but absent in 15 to 23 percent of those Americans over 50.

Sugar, which has been linked to heart disease (and will be discussed in Chapter 20), causes a severe consumption of chromium. Dr. Schroeder has shown that 150 grams (or 5 ounces) of white sugar would cause a net loss of 12 to 25 micrograms of chromium in the urine in a single day, or about 8.75 milligrams in a single year, more than the total body content. The loss of chromium occurs because as soon as sugar is eaten, chromium pours into the bloodstream, after which most of it is lost to the urine.

Natural sources of chromium are whole wheat, peas, and brewer's yeast. Chelated chromium or yeast is the preferred form as a normal ingredient in your multivitamin and mineral formulations.

As modern processed foods become more and more refined, the traces of zinc, copper, and chromium provided by nature are disappearing from our diets. Over long periods of time, these small losses of trace minerals can lead to large problems, such as heart disease. Returned to the diet over a long period of administration, these trace minerals can help heal the heart and arteries.

18

Don't Drink the Water If It's Chlorinated

Our bodies have little need for chlorine. (Chlorine used for water purification is a "bleaching" *gas,* and is not to be confused with chloride, which is part of the table-salt molecule.) Someday we will stop forcing so many chlorinated chemicals into ourselves via drinking water. The EPA has detected a number of chlorinated carcinogens in the drinking water of several American cities. Yet that is only half the picture. There is evidence that chlorine and many chlorinated compounds can cause the monoclonal cell proliferation that forms the plaques in arteries. In addition to its mutagenic action, chlorine destroys the protective vitamin E.

Many municipalities are unaware of the benefits of ozone (a form of oxygen) for water purification and the disadvantages of chlorine. Only those people drinking well water, spring water, or carbon-filtered water escape the harm of chlorine. Recently, several companies have introduced inexpensive screw-on gadgets for the kitchen water faucet that remove chlorine and other pollutants by carbon filtering. The carbon filters make the water taste better and make it safer. (I will not give my dog tap water without carbon filtration.)

Chlorinated Water Correlates with Increased Rate of Heart Disease

A small-scale study by Ronald Pataki (a colleague of mine in Jersey City, N.J.) found that Jersey City people over 50 years of age having heart disease drank tap water in quantities correlating with the severity of their disease. And he found that those over 50 years of age not having heart disease drank either bottled water, boiled water, or mostly other fluids. (Boiling water releases the chlorine, which bubbles out as gas in the steam.)

The differences in heart-disease death rates between groups in comparisons such as the Boston-Irish Brothers study or the Northern-Southern Indian study could be explained in terms of chlorine. The brothers who live in Ireland and had the low heart-disease rate were still drinking chlorine-free water at the time of the study. Now that their homes are receiving chlorinated water, the heart-disease death rate may soon increase. In south India, the water is chlorinated, but in north India, where water is not generally chlorinated, there is less heart disease. Since the water of the capital city, New Delhi, in the north has been chlorinated, the heart-disease death rate there has begun to climb.

Even small but growing American towns like Roseto, Pennsylvania (which until recently had an uncommonly low incidence of heart disease), have experienced increasing heart-disease death rates—possibly because newcomers and the younger-generation families rely on tap water rather than the spring water that the oldtimers drink.

Doctors Warn against Chlorine

Dr. Herbert Schwartz (of Cumberland County College in Vineland, N.J.) believes that chlorine has so many dangers it should be banned. He has told the EPA that "putting chlorine in the water is like starting a time bomb."

Dr. Joseph Price (of Saginaw General Hospital in Michigan) told reporter James Quinlan that "chlorine is the cause of an unprecedented disease epidemic which includes heart attacks and strokes. Chlorine is an insidious poison. Most medical researchers were led to believe it was safe, but we are now learning the hard way that all the time we thought we were preventing epidemics of one disease, we were creating another. Two decades after the start of chlorinating our drinking water in 1904, the present epidemic of heart trouble and cancer began." (*National Enquirer,* December 24, 1974.)

Dr. Price tested the effects of chlorine on chickens and found all the chickens receiving chlorinated water showed evidence of either atherosclerosis of the aorta or obstruction of the circulatory system. He has written a book on the subject which you will find helpful if you are interested in pursuing the chlorine–heart-disease relationship further— *Coronaries, Cholesterol, Chlorine* (Pyramid, 1974).

Dr. Robert Carlson of the University of Minnesota points out that "when chlorine is used to treat water, it doesn't disappear. It shows up in thousands of new compounds that it reacts with."

If you still have doubts about the harmful effects of chlorine, consider the situation in Japan. Japan abandoned chlorination after the post–World War II occupation by American troops—and their heart-disease death rate is currently about one-sixth of ours.

19

Special Food Supplements: Lecithin, Garlic, Yogurt, and Bran

There are no magic foods for the prevention of heart disease. However, there are foods rich in the nutrients often lacking in our diets. A deficiency of any nutrient hampers the body in its effort to stay healthy and normal, and heart disease can be one of the results of a deficiency of even a single nutrient. If your present diet is not well-rounded, you may wish to balance it by adding rich sources of the missing nutrients. **Remember, all the nutrients are not yet known, so just taking vitamin and mineral pills won't guarantee optimum nutrition. A highly diversified diet, supplemented by vitamins and minerals to compensate for the nutrients lost during food processing and storage, is essential, and the inclusion of some food concentrates (known as food supplements) is often wise.**

High Lecithin Levels Correlate Well with Lack of Atherosclerosis

Lecithin (pronounced *less*-e-thin) has long been a staple for nutrition-conscious people concerned with lowering their blood cholesterol levels. When nourished properly, the body makes all the lecithin it needs, but if certain key nutrients such as vitamin B$_6$, magnesium, choline (a B-complex vitamin), and polyunsaturated fatty acids are missing, then the body's lecithin production will be inadequate.

Although lecithin has been in popular use to make cholesterol soluble in the bloodstream, its role in preventing heart disease is twofold.

First, lecithin's chief value may be in maintaining membrane integrity, the formation of prostaglandins (hormone-like chemicals), blood-pressure control, and platelet health. (As an essential component of membranes, lecithin provides the phospholipids required for the membrane bi-layer of red blood cells that provides the polar charge that keeps red blood cells apart.)

Second, a deficiency causes abnormal fat transport in the artery walls (because the enzyme lecithin-cholesterol acyltransferase cannot be manufacturered in adequate amounts). Abnormal fat transport can cause a variety of problems for the body.

A report by Dr. F. S. van Buchem (of the Netherlands) revealed that men having lecithin levels above 36 percent of total blood fats had *no* signs of atherosclerosis or related diseases, even though many of those men had high blood cholesterol levels. On the other hand, the men having lecithin levels less than 34 percent of total blood fat *all* had some signs of heart disease (*Nutrition,* 1962).

When a deficiency of lecithin exists, the body cannot function properly: membranes are weakened, arteries develop abnormalities, and prostaglandins are not produced in normal amounts. Over 20 years ago, it was found that experimental rats on a lecithin-deficient diet developed either cardiac degeneration or renal (kidney) lesions (C.H. Best, *Science,* 1954).

An easy way to ensure that you have the nutrients required for lecithin production is to eat foods rich in lecithin (such as egg yolks, milk, and soybeans) or take supplements of lecithin itself. As a food supplement, which may be taken straight or in food, one or two tablespoons (6 to 12 grams) daily is adequate. Up to three times that much (36 grams) has reduced the pain of angina. Be advised, however, that there are 110 calories in each tablespoon. The use of lecithin in curing atherosclerosis will be detailed in Chapter

31, in which Dr. Jacobus Rinse, a retired physician now living in Vermont, describes how to combine various special supplements to cure heart disease.

Garlic Normalizes Blood Pressure

Some foods do appear to have special medicinal properties, even though they do not act specifically as a medicine against heart disease. Honey and garlic, for example, have sterile properties. Because molds cannot grow in honey, Russian surgeons often prescribe it prior to surgery in an attempt to prevent infections.

Garlic also has been shown to kill bacteria in the bloodstream; hence it has been widely known as a blood purifier. Nobel Prize Laureate Dr. Arthur Stoll established in the 1940s the antibiotic effect of garlic and ascribed this power to the alliin (a sulfur-containing amino acid) present in garlic.

About 25 years later, garlic was found to destroy the bacteria E-coli and salmonella. Biochemist Dr. C. Edward Burtis attributed the antibioticlike effect to garlic's stimulation of glandular activity.

The blood-purification properties of garlic are not especially significant with respect to heart disease. I mention them to keep the record straight and to illustrate that, since foods contain several compounds (some nutrients in nature or function, some pharmacological, and others inert), some foods are capable of several functions.

Garlic, like vitamin E, reduces blood-platelet adhesion. It also normalizes blood pressure in some people, and has prevented normal atherosclerotic plaques in some laboratory animals.

Plaque prevention attributed to garlic supplements in experimental rabbits on high-cholesterol diets was demonstrated by pathologist Dr. R.C. Jain (of the University of Benghazi in Libya) and reported in *Lancet,* 1975. Reduction of blood-platelet adhesion resulting from garlic supplements in humans was shown by Drs. Arun Bordia and H.C.

Bansal (of R.N.T. Medical College, Udaipur, India) following which it was reported in *Lancet,* 1973. (Remember from Chapter 3 that platelet adhesion is the first step in forming the clot that causes a coronary, and that lowering the platelet-adhesion index to normal is beneficial.)

Garlic is rich in selenium, and I believe that it's the selenium that's effective in preventing platelet adhesion and clot formation, as well as high blood pressure, and not the other components of garlic. Selenium has also been shown to protect people against infections. (See Chapter 11.)

Garlic can be conveniently added to your daily diet in capsule form, which doesn't leave you with garlic breath. For those who enjoy the taste, fresh garlic adds zest to any meat or meat sandwich, including hamburger. If fresh garlic doesn't suit your taste, substitute onions, or make sure you eat other foods rich in selenium (such as tuna and eggs) every week.

The fact that in 1971 Italians (whose cooking often contains garlic) had less than one-third of the U.S. heart-disease death rate is an interesting observation. (Note Table 2.3.) For years race horse trainers have fed garlic to race horses to prevent atherosclerosis.

Yogurt Lowers Blood Cholesterol Levels

Yogurt is perhaps the most widely recognized special food among health-food advocates. It's been around for centuries, and some of the most long-lived people in the world (Turks, Bulgarians, and Russians living in the Caucasus) eat it.

Although the medical establishment has never believed that yogurt possessed medicinal properties, it has been found by Dr. G. U. Mann (Associate Professor of Biochemistry and Medicine at Vanderbilt University) to contain an ingredient that reduces cholesterol levels in people, even when their diet is high in cholesterol. Peoples such as the Maasai (East African people whose diet is rich in yogurt) have almost no heart disease. I attribute this to their abundance of physical activity and their balance between calories eaten and calories expended. The relationship between blood cholesterol levels and heart disease is not as significant as either calorie balance or physical activity. (See Chapter 26.)

However, yogurt can lower blood cholesterol levels even among people consuming excess calories and putting on weight. This is exactly what happened among the Maasai taking part in an experiment conducted by Dr. Mann. Although the Maasai in the study overate, because the yogurt was provided at no cost, their already low blood cholesterol levels (135) dropped even lower. Later Dr. Mann repeated the test on adult Americans and noted the same drastic reduction in blood cholesterol (*American Journal of Clinical Nutrition,* 1975). It may be that the bacteria that ferments the milk into yogurt affects the liver's production of cholesterol.

Be advised, however, that there is at least one report that associates an entire diet of commercial yogurt with eye cataracts in animals. The quantity tested was fed to experimental rats as their sole source of food, and the issue remains unsettled at this time, although another experiment by the same researcher with home-made yogurt did not produce cataracts. If the findings do hold up, the culprit may well be a chemical used in large-scale commercial production.

Bran and Alfalfa—High-Fiber Supplements

Because it's desirable to have adequate roughage in our diet, especially since foods are becoming more and more refined and overprocessed, eating starchy vegetables and whole grains is especially important. Supplements that are relatively high in bulk are bran and alfalfa (both of which contain B-complex vitamins and minerals). Bran is from grain, and whole grains include the bran. Bran and alfalfa can be bought at health-food stores and in some supermarkets.

Foods play a major part in the prevention of heart disease.

Sometime it's the nutrients we miss that lead to heart disease. We can return those nutrients to our bodies and improve our health by adding lecithin-rich foods, garlic, onions, yogurt, bran, and alfalfa to our diets. In Chapter 31, several ways of combining these special food supplements into pleasant-tasting meals, including Dr. Rinse's Breakfast, are given.

20

Life Is Sweeter without Sugar

Much has been said in recent years concerning the dangers of sugar in our refined diets. Yet, food processors and consumers alike insist on the removal of unrefined carbohydrates from their foods and the substitution of refined sugar. The ratio of complex to refined sugars in the American diet has changed from nearly 3 to 1 in 1889 to (2 to 1 in 1909, almost 1 to 1 in 1932) to less than 1 to 1 in 1961 (M. Antar et al., *American Journal of Clinical Nutrition,* 1964).

The biggest problem with sugar is that it has been added to so many foods that we eat relatively large quantities of it every day (equivalent to 35 teaspoons or about 350 calories daily, or one pound every three days). (H. J. Roberts, *Journal of the American Geriatric Society,* 1967.) Dr. Emanuel Cheraskin has estimated that refined sugar is present in 90 percent of our retail foods (E. Cheraskin, W. Ringsdorf, and A. Brecher, *Psychodietetics,* Stein and Day, 1974). The average consumption of sugar is 105 pounds per person per year; 150 years ago, Americans ate 3 pounds per year. You may not even know when you are eating sugar, but in nearly every processed food it's there to boost both flavor and sales.

Refined Sugar Destroys Nutrients

Refined sugar consumes vitamins and minerals, particularly vitamin B_6 and chromium. These nutrients are critical to a healthy heart, and unless the body has excess stores of each, the average sugar intake will cause a deficiency of each and eventually a weakened heart. If you eat processed foods, you must be sure your diet is rich in B-complex and chromium. (See Chapters 13 and 17.)

If you are certain your diet is rich in B vitamins and chromium, there is little harm in having an occasional sweet. But the problem with eating more than an occasional sweet is that refined sugar throws the body's appetite control out of whack, and you can easily develop a craving for more sweets. When you're tempted by sweets, remember that a statistical relationship does exist between the incidence of heart disease, the consumption of total calories, and obesity.

Older People Require Fewer Calories

The older you get, the more important it becomes to get your nutrients in the fewest calories possible. As we age, our bodies develop a slower metabolism and require fewer calories to carry out the life processes. Additionally, we generally decrease our physical activity as time goes by, again burning fewer calories, with the excess converted to fat. If we cut back on our calories, yet waste some of the few calories on sugar, we limit the amount of nutrients we take in. If we make sure we get our nutrients, yet still include sugar in our diets, we may consume too many calories and become fatter. Either way, with sweets we lose.

Let's look at some of the reasons researchers have been linking sugar consumption to heart disease.

Dietary Sugar Is a Greater Problem Than Dietary Fat

Dr. Richard A. Ahrens (of the Food, Nutrition, and Institution Administration Department of the University of Maryland) sees dietary sugar as a far greater problem than dietary fat. In a review of sugar, hypertension, and heart disease, Dr. Ahrens concluded: "The most carefully designed studies have consistently shown that heart disease victims do consume more sugar; although there have been differences in the size of this difference and several have tried to 'explain it away' by attributing the heart disease to the higher consumption of coffee or cigarettes in the group eating the most sugar. It is relevant to observe that the pandemic of heart disease continues to increase on a worldwide scale in rough proportion to the increase in sugar consumption, but not in proportion with saturated fat intake." (*American Journal of Clinical Nutrition,* 1974.)

Dr. John Yudkin (Emeritus Professor of Nutrition at London University) found that the most striking dietary change in Western nations during the heart-disease epidemic has been the seven-fold increase in the consumption of refined sugar. Dr. Yudkin pointed out that the wealthier nations with the highest incidence of heart disease also consume the most sugar. He further observed that the sugar consumption of heart-disease victims was higher prior to their first heart attack than the sugar consumption of carefully matched control subjects free of heart disease (*Proceedings of the Nutrition Society,* 1964).

Similar reports from Czechoslovakia and South Africa also show that sugar intakes were highest in those groups having the highest incidence of heart disease (K. Oscanova, *American Journal of Clinical Nutrition,* 1967; A.R.P. Walker, *Journal of South African Medicine,* 1968).

How Sugar Can Cause Heart Disease

Dr. A. A. Gigon (of Germany) has shown that adding sugar to adequate diets causes many species of animals to malnourish themselves to the point of death. Additionally, sugar increases blood pressure (Ahrens, 1974), and elevates blood levels of triglycerides (J. I. Mann et al., *Clinical Sciences,* 1971). A number of animal studies have concluded that replacing starch calories with sugar calories shortens the average lifespan (I. MacDonald and G. A. Thomas, *Clinical Sciences,* 1956; A. M. Durand et al., *Ar-*

chieves of Pathology, 1968; L. M. Dalderup and W. Visser, *Nature,* 1969).

Other researchers have pinpointed the excessive ingestion of sugar to hyperinsulinism and diabetes mellitus. Diabetes is a valid risk factor in heart disease, and diabetics often have abnormal blood platelets which cause blood clotting. Dr. Yudkin has shown that high sugar consumption causes increased blood-platelet stickiness (*Nature,* 1972). Earlier we emphasized that it is the increased blood-platelet adhesion that has caused the epidemic of heart-disease deaths. It was noted that plaques in the arteries alone would not cause death, and that vitamin E reduced the chances of clotting by normalizing the blood-platelet adhesion index.

There is evidence that eating foods rich in sugar can bring on angina pains and even cause heart attacks because the sugary meal results in the overproduction of insulin and a sharp fall in the blood sugar levels (Dr. Benjamin P. Sandler, *Internal Medicine News,* 1974).

In the 1974 British report on diet and coronary heart disease, Dr. Yudkin emphasized the association of heart disease and the sugar-insulin diseases of diabetes and hypoglycemia:

"Although the role of insulin may be secondary, it is relevant to point out that increased physical activity, which reduces the risk of heart disease, reduces the blood concentration of insulin [which is desirable]. On the other hand, obesity, diabetes, peripheral vascular disease and cigarette smoking, all of which are associated with heart disease, are found to produce increased concentrations of blood insulin. This effect they share with dietary sugar."

Stress is another risk factor in heart disease, and our ability to deal with stress is reduced by excess sugar in the diet. The sudden fall in blood sugar level that occurs about three hours after a high-sugar meal makes a person irritable. Dr. E. Cheraskin says, "By far the biggest culprit in the inability to deal with stress is refined sugar. If you reduce your sugar intake, you will notice an incredible change in your personality. It will be much easier to conquer stress situations that previously caused bad temper and impatience."

On several fronts, refined sugar is our sweet enemy.

Sugar leads to many body upsets, any one of which could lead to artery and heart disease. Diabetes has long been recognized as a risk factor in heart disease, but the metabolic upsets caused by hypoglycemia have been ignored as a cause. Hypoglycemia is a condition that causes low blood sugar. I cannot offer you experimental evidence specifically linking hypoglycemia with heart disease, but it is my opinion that the statistical link between sugar consumption and heart disease has its highest correlation among those individuals suffering from diabetes and hypoglycemia. Patients given a low-sugar diet for hypoglycemia experience fewer angina attacks.

The two most important books that have been published on hypoglycemia are *Low Blood Sugar and You* by Carlton Fredericks, Ph.D., and Herman Goodman, M.D., (Constellation International, 1969) which has helped many thousands of people, including my brother, Stanley Passwater, and *Nutrigenetics* by R. O. Brennan, M.D., and W. C. Mulligan (Evans, 1975). *Nutrigenetics* relates thirty years of experience in controlling hypoglycemia and preventing the degenerative diseases that normally follow—including diabetes, heart disease, stroke, and liver and kidney disease. Other excellent books on the subject include *Psychodietetics, Megavitamin Therapy,* and *Hypoglycemia.* See Suggested Readings for details.

21
It's Rougher without Roughage

The current interest in roughage stems from further research on a discovery by Nobel Laureate Dr. Denis Burkitt.
What Dr. Burkitt realized was that bowel cancer is essentially unknown in Uganda among those Africans eating their
native high-bulk diet. Dr. Burkitt, who was a surgeon in
Uganda for 20 years and is now a member of Britain's Medical Research Council, found that the residue from the high-
fiber diet was eliminated from the bowel in less than half
the time required by the residue of the refined Western
diets (35 hours for the Africans, 77–100 hours for English-
men). This relatively speedy elimination, I believe, may prevent a buildup of degradation products (which are dangerous free-radical producers).

Another advantage of "crude" diets is that they release
carbohydrates slowly rather than abruptly as refined sugar
does, and, consequently, the insulin-glucose balance isn't
upset. The bulk is also filling and reduces hunger.

Additional studies of the African diet and health revealed
that although many African diets are high in cholesterol (see
Chapters 4 and 5), the incidence of coronary thrombosis is
essentially nil. Further investigation by several scientists
linked the high-fiber diet to increased production of bile
acids which were formed from cholesterol. Also, the bulk
reduces the amount of bile acids reabsorbed by the large
intestine. Thus, the presence of bulk in the bowel removes
cholesterol from the bloodstream.

This is reassuring if you believe the cholesterol theory.

However, this doesn't explain why additional cholesterol is not manufacturered by the body to replace the consumed cholesterol. Little mention is made of the fact that people in this country have heart attacks even though their blood cholesterol levels are as low as the Africans'.

I believe a high-fiber diet helps prevent heart disease, but not because it consumes cholesterol. In Chapter 3, it was explained that heart disease, like cancer, was caused by free radicals which encourage cells to grow wildly. In the case of heart disease, smooth muscle cells in the artery wall are mutated by the free radicals (formed as a result of food degradation in the bowel, and by cigarette smoke and other pollutants). The monoclonal proliferation of the mutated cells leads to plaques which, at a later stage of development, produce their own cholesterol and collagen. Finally, the plaques erupt into the bloodstream and at each such location the collagen becomes a site for clot formation.

Besides producing fewer free radicals, the African native diet is rich in antioxidant nutrients which our society refines out of its food supply. To prevent heart disease, Americans must do more than eat high-fiber diets; they must also replace the antioxidants—vitamin E and selenium.

High-Fiber Foods

One good way to increase your dietary fiber is to reduce or stop eating junk foods (usually refined white flour and refined white sugar) and start eating more fresh fruits and vegetables.

If you consult food tables in an attempt to find high-fiber foods, it's helpful to know that such tables generally list crude fiber (CF) which is the remaining portion of food resistant to treatment with boiling acid. This differs slightly from dietary fiber (DF), the portion of plant cells that are resistant to hydrolysis (breakup) by the enzymes of man. Only one-fifth to one-half of the total dietary fiber is actually crude fiber, but still crude fiber is a good index by which to judge the bulk content of foods.

Typical Western diets contain 5–6 grams of crude fiber daily, in contrast to typical "native" diets containing 23–25 grams. Our intake of fresh fruit and vegetables has declined from an annual average of 250 pounds per person in 1940 to an annual average of less than 180 pounds per person in 1970. Meanwhile, the consumption of processed fruit and vegetables has increased from a yearly average of 65 pounds per person in 1940 to 110 pounds per person in 1970.

If the foods were of equivalent value, this would indicate, on the average, an annual decrease in the consumption of fruits and vegetables of 25 pounds per person; but we are receiving proportionately far less because dietary fiber is largely removed from processed foods. Additionally, the fiber consumption from whole grains has decreased by 50 percent during the first half of the twentieth century.

Several researchers have recommended taking 2 teaspoons of unprocessed miller's bran with each meal. Bran tablets are also available. But the best plan is to add whole grains and fresh fruits and vegetables to your diet. Popular high-fiber foods are potatoes (including skins), rice bran, tapioca starch, rolled oats, whole-grain breads, whole fruits (including skins), lettuce, celery, carrots, corn, popcorn, apples, alfalfa, kelp, and any leafy vegetable. "An apple a day keeps the doctor away" is a more apt maxim today than it was when it was coined.

22

The Number That Counts—
Your Blood Pressure

Your present blood pressure is perhaps the most important number you can know. If it's high, you had best not ignore it. High blood pressure is the leading contributing cause of death in Western countries today, helping to kill "1 out of 8 of everybody who will die from anything." (U.S. Government document No. NIH 74–681.)

This year alone, high blood pressure will help kill 250,000 Americans. That's five times as many people as are killed each year in automobile accidents. Fortunately, high blood pressure takes a long time to do its lethal damage, and it responds well to treatment. Unfortunately, half of the people who have it don't know it, and if you don't know about it, you can't treat it. What's your blood pressure today?

When Dr. Charles C. Edwards was the Assistant Secretary of Health, Education, and Welfare, he repeatedly warned that high blood pressure is our most neglected killer. He emphasized that about 12 million people with high blood pressure don't even know that they are harboring this insidious disease and that even millions more who are aware of their high blood pressure skip lifesaving treatment perhaps hoping that if they ignore it, it will go away. But high blood pressure doesn't work that way. Dr. Edwards estimated that 24 million Americans, including one of every seven adults, had high blood pressure in 1974, but that only 10 to 20 percent received adequate treatment.

Yet, high blood pressure is directly responsible for

60,000 deaths a year and is indirectly responsible for more than one-quarter of the million deaths annually from stroke and cardiovascular disease.

Dr. Edwards stressed that there is no such thing as "benign hypertension" (once taught in medical school to be a harmless form of high blood pressure), and that even a slight elevation in pressure is a risk factor that can lead to a variety of health problems including heart attack, stroke, blindness, and kidney failure.

Most people with high blood pressure are unaware of their condition because they have no symptoms and may even feel fine. They are not even nervous or tense, as many people believe you are with high blood pressure. The medical name for high blood pressure is hypertension, but that doesn't mean that you have to be tense in order to get it.

Other people do have symptoms that warn them. Frequent signs of high blood pressure include one or more of the following: dizziness, ringing in ears, headaches, tiredness, nosebleeds, red streaks in the eye whites, unexplained aches and pains, swollen ankles, heart palpitations, frequent urination, and crossness. Some of these symptoms are vague and can be caused by several problems or even be of harmless origins, so don't assume you have or do not have high blood pressure—get it measured and know for sure.

Don't ignore opportunities to find out what your blood pressure is. Get in the habit of asking what it is when the doctor takes it, or better yet, learn to take it yourself. Blood pressure normally goes up and down with emotion, fear, excitement, etc.; so don't rely on one measurement. It's a problem only when the pressure is consistently high.

Some people have occasional spurts of high blood pressure during bursts of anger or stress, and they can feel the pulse in their temples and feel their faces turn warm and red. Yet this occasional stress-response increase in blood pressure seems to be perfectly harmless.

As Dr. Theodore Cooper (former Director of the National Heart, Lung, and Blood Institute) summed it up in Dr. Frank Finnerty's excellent book, *High Blood Pressure* (McKay,

1975), "Few people, if given a choice, would choose to die young. Fewer would choose to live out their lives crippled, blind, or unable to think or speak clearly. Yet, this is the fate of many people with high blood pressure. It is a burden doubly hard to bear because it is unnecessary. Most of the complications can be prevented in most people. Certainly, the appearance of complications can be postponed."

Table 22.1

Blood Pressure and Life Expectancy

Age	Blood Pressure	Added Life Expectancy (years)	
		Men	Women
35	120/80	41.5	?
	130/90	37.5	?
	140/95	32.5	?
	150/100	25	?
45	120/80	32	37
	130/90	29	35.5
	140/95	26	32
	150/100	20.5	28.5
55	120/80	23.5	27.5
	130/90	22.5	27
	140/95	19.5	24.5
	150/100	17.5	23.5

(Courtesy Metropolitan Life Insurance Company)

Life insurance companies rely heavily on blood-pressure measurement as their most important factor predicting life expectancy. Isn't it about time you did? (See Table 22.1.)

High Diastolic Pressure Is Dangerous

The fact that reduction of high blood pressure is actually beneficial and practical has been established by Dr. Edward D. Freis of the Veterans Hospital in Washington.

In 1963, Dr. Freis and his colleagues studied 523 men in 17 VA hospitals. All 523 men were selected because they had moderately high blood pressure with the bottom number, called the diastolic, between 90 and 130. Previously, medical schools had taught that it would not do men in this blood-pressure range much good to have their pressure normalized.

During the study, the men were divided into two groups with about half (the experimental group) getting blood-pressure-lowering drugs, and the remainder (the control group) receiving sugar pills (placebos).

After 16 months, 143 control-group patients with diastolic blood pressure over 115 were withdrawn from the study because their health was in jeopardy. During these first 16 months, four of the untreated patients (receiving only the placebos) died, and 23 others in that group developed serious complications. In contrast, among those receiving effective medication, there were no deaths and only 2 serious complications.

The remainder, the 380 with diastolics between 90 and 115, were periodically checked for a total time in excess of 5 years. The dramatic results showed the death rate of the treated group was only half the death rate of the untreated group. Furthermore, those in the treated group had only one-third (18 percent vs. 55 percent) the number of serious complications.

Clearly, for those with high diastolic blood pressure, prolonged drug treatment can be worthwhile. Yet many people, if not most, can normalize their blood pressure without drugs. Nutrition and biofeedback can both be used to cure or control blood pressure without the need for drugs or, at least, with smaller amounts of drugs required. Just reducing body weight is all that is necessary for many.

Some blood-pressure-control drugs have serious side

effects ranging from cancer to sexual impotence. Fortunately, there are over 50 drugs to choose from, so that the harmful drugs can be avoided. The reason there are so many drugs is that the cause of high blood pressure is not well understood, so there is no specific drug to treat it. Before we look at nutritional control of blood pressure and drugs with adverse side effects, let's look at the origin of high blood pressure.

The Cause and Effect of High Blood Pressure

When the heart pumps blood through the body, the blood passes through arteries, arterioles, capillaries, and returns through veins. The important part of the circulatory loop is the arteriole system (the smallest branches of an artery before it becomes a capillary). These arterioles regulate blood pressure more than any other body part. Arterioles control blood pressure by controlling the ease or difficulty with which the pumped blood can get to the capillaries. (An arteriole can be likened to a nozzle that regulates water pressure in a hose.) The arterioles have muscular overcoats controlled by the automatic nervous system—which, itself, is not fully understood (although it is know that part of the regulation is by prostaglandins and the enzyme renin).

When the heart beats, blood is pumped into the arteries, which stretch slightly to accommodate the surge of blood. The maximum pressure in the arteries is at the moment of the heart beat and is the first number (called systolic) reported in your blood-pressure measurement. After the beat, the blood surges through the circulatory system, but remains under pressure in the arteries, because another surge of blood pushes against it with the next beat. (If the heart stopped, the pressure in arteries and veins would fall to zero.) Thus, the pressure reaches a maximum at the beat, then falls while the heart rests until the lowest figure in the blood pressure measurement (called diastolic) is reached, at which point it starts to rise as the heart beats again. The measurement of the pressure is expressed in millimeters of mercury, representing the height to which a column of mercury will be pushed by that pressure.

Factors that affect the blood pressure include the control of the arterioles, the amount of tissue (fat) that must be serviced by the heart, the elasticity and diameter of the arteries, the excess pressure of water in the tissues or increased blood volume due to water retention, the health of the kidney, smoking, or taking birth-control pills. (Yes, one in four women on "the pill" develops high blood pressure.)

When the heart has to work harder to pump blood through the body because of high blood pressure, it can become enlarged and less elastic. The pressure can damage the retina and optic nerve or rupture an artery. The arteries also may become less elastic and release chemicals into the bloodstream that can cause the monoclonal proliferation that leads to heart disease. (See Chapters 2 and 3.)

These same chemicals that cause monoclonal proliferation *may* also be responsible for the threefold increase in the cancer rate observed in men with high blood pressure. A study by Dr. Alan R. Dyer (biostatistician at Northwestern University Medical School) analyzed the relationship between high blood pressure and cancer in 1,233 men over a 14-year period. The men who had high blood pressure at the time of their 1958 exams were about three times as likely to die from cancer as men with normal blood pressure. By 1972, 246 of the men had died, 71 from cancer. This does not prove cause and effect, but it does pinpoint a trend that needs further study.

How High Is "High"?

Since the study by Dr. Freis, physicians now take a new look at both diastolic and systolic levels in determing whether you have high blood pressure. Before Freis's report, many physicians had accepted the old rule of thumb that normal or acceptable blood pressure was 100 plus your age. (This of course referred to the systolic measurement, the first and higher reading.)

The old rule is certainly incorrect, as shown by Dr. Freis's study. Your blood pressure should be or controlled to be the level you had at 20 or 21 years of age. A good reading is 110/70. Freis says anything over 120/80 is not good and 160/95 is serious. Figures 22.1 and 22.2 show the spread of blood-pressure values according to age and sex in the U.S. Medical researchers today feel that it's the diastolic pressure that's most important.

Previously, high blood pressure was defined as "essential hypertension" if its cause was unknown, which was the situation in 90 to 95 percent of all cases of sustained (prolonged) high blood pressure. "Essential" didn't mean that it

Figure 22.1 Percent distribution of systolic blood pressure of the population 18–74 years by age and sex: United States, 1971–72
From USDHEW Publication No. HRA 75–1632

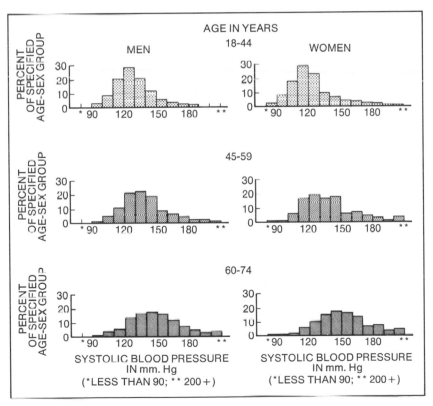

was necessary; it was medical language for "without known cause." Today the term "primary high blood pressure" is replacing the term "essential hypertension." The terms "benign" and "malignant" have also been discarded, basically because there is no such thing as "benign" high blood pressure.

Many doctors now follow the three categories of the New York Heart Association as a guide. "Borderline hypertension" refers to blood pressures with systolic levels between 140 and 160 accompanied by diastolic levels between 90

Figure 22.2 Percent distribution of diastolic blood pressure of the population 18–74 years by age and sex: United States, 1971–72
From USDHEW Publication No. HRA 75–1632

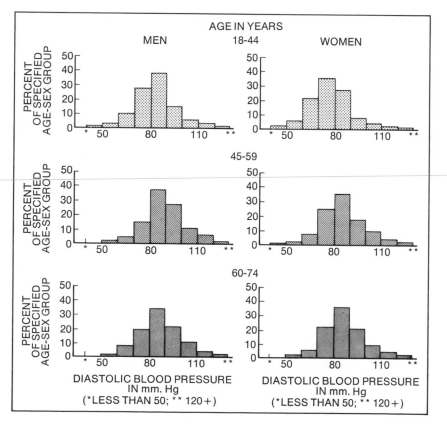

and 95."Moderate hypertension" refers to systolics between 160 and 180 with diastolics between 90 and 95. "Marked hypertension" refers to systolics above 180 or diastolics above 115. (120/90 or 130/90 would be okay, according to NYSHA standards, but would bear watching—although not yet in the gray zone or danger zone.)

The World Health Organization protocols classify blood pressures below 140/90 as normal, and 180/95 as hypertensive, with the in-between "gray zone" subject to interpretation.

The National Health Survey of 1962 had defined hypertension to include either or both a systolic of 160 or higher, or a diastolic of 95 or higher.

Free Blood-Pressure Screening Programs

As the American Heart Association says, "Perform a death-defying act—have your blood pressure checked." Yes, you can defy death by learning your blood pressure and controlling it if it's elevated. But how do you find out what your blood pressure is? Simple—call your local chapter of the American Heart Association and ask where the nearest free screening center is. If there is no local chapter of the AHA where you live, call the health or safety officer where you work, or call the public health service or the nearest hospital for information about free screening programs. Every time you visit your doctor, ask what your blood pressure is. Many dentists are even screening their patients in an effort to locate those at risk.

Checking Your Own Blood Pressure

The best program, however, is to take your blood pressure yourself. Buy a sphygmomanometer (the instrument for measuring blood pressure) and a stethoscope (the instrument for listening to the heart and lungs) from a drugstore, mail-order catalog, or health-food magazine. Stethoscopes generally cost $3 to $10. Sphygmomanometers typically sell for about $20 to $25, but can range up to $40. These are good investments that may help keep someone with marked high blood pressure from dying 20 years prematurely.

Taking your own blood pressure is easier than saying "sphygmomanometer." Detailed instructions come with the instrument, and, basically, the procedure involves wrapping a cloth cuff around the biceps and pumping air into the cuff with a rubber bulb which inflates the cuff.

When the pressure in the cuff becomes greater than the blood pressure in the brachial artery of the arm, the flow of blood is temporarily stopped, because the squeeze of the cuff is greater than the push of the blood in the artery. The stethoscope, which has been pressed against the forearm just below the inside of the elbow, confirms that the blood flow has ceased when the heartbeat is no longer heard. Now you are ready to measure the blood pressure.

The valve in the air bulb is turned slightly so that the air in the cuff can be released slowly. When the air pressure in the cuff drops just slightly below the level of the systolic pressure in the brachial artery, the beat of the heart can be heard. Right at that point you record the measurement for the systolic pressure.

Continue to let the air out of the cuff until the distinct heartbeat sound disappears. At that point, record the diastolic pressure.

Generally the pulse gets louder after the systolic pressure and then fades until the diastolic pressure is reached. At this point the blood is flowing steadily through the artery and no beat is heard.

When you first start taking your own blood pressure, expect the readings to be a little high. The anxiety of taking the measurement is enough to raise the blood pressure. Often a doctor will repeat the measurement because of this anxiety, and the second reading is usually appreciably lower than the first. Don't try to take more than two readings at a time because the reliability of the measurement decreases with all that disturbance on the brachial artery.

To find your blood-pressure pattern, take your blood pressure twice a day for a week, and then daily until you are sure that you have found your average blood pressure. Some people will note blood-pressure cycles and patterns and they should try to discover the causes of the variance. Once your average or pattern has been ascertained, readings should be taken monthly. Any sustained increase of 10 points or more is reason to see your doctor (but not cause for alarm).

Most likely an increase in blood pressure will parallel recent weight gains, and shedding a few pounds will return your pressure to normal. Unfortunately, all increases in blood pressure aren't due to weight gains. If this were true, skinny people would be free of high blood pressure. Dr. Paul Podmajersky (a Las Vegas bariatric physician, or obesity specialist) estimates that 76 percent of U.S. adults are overweight, have high blood pressure, or both. Therefore, three out of four should lose some weight for both reasons.

Even if you only use your sphygmomanometer once a month for each adult member of the household, it is a fantastic investment. It lasts indefinitely and is the best indicator of health around. It detects trouble before you can feel any difference, and early treatment brings outstanding results. While you are taking your blood pressure, record your pulse as well. Keep a log of both your blood pressure and pulse. Figure 32.2 provides a convenient chart on which to record your blood pressure for your physician's interpretation.

If your blood pressure is elevated, you should take more frequent readings than indicated in the total protection plan (Figure 32.2). More frequent readings may help your physician spot trends that can lead to the control of your blood pressure.

Control Your High Blood Pressure

The three main weapons against high blood pressure are diet, drugs, and biofeedback. Exercise and the reduction of smoking and stress are also effective measures.

Dietary control is the preferred method when you first notice an increase in blood pressure, and it can be effective alone or with medication. If diet doesn't bring the desired normalization within two to three months, see your doctor and start mild medication. If your blood pressure is markedly elevated, use diet, drugs, and biofeedback simultaneously.

If you have elevated blood pressure, read on. The following chapter will tell you specifically how to control it, with or without drugs.

23

Controlling Blood Pressure, with and without Drugs

The dietary weapons for use against high blood pressure include weight reduction; salt restriction; and vitamin E, selenium, vitamin B$_{15}$, potassium, lecithin, and garlic supplements. Any one of these weapons may work for you, or a combination may be required. Because each person is biochemically unique and there are many possible causes of high blood pressure, your task is to find which weapon or combination will cure or control your high blood pressure.

Losing Weight Can Save Your Life

First of all, stand in front of a mirror. Do you see flab? Can you grab a handful? Ordinarily that might be harmless, but if you have high blood pressure, your excess weight becomes deadly. With high blood pressure, you are the one in ten who has to watch your weight. A mile of capillaries (literally) is required to nourish each extra pound of tissue. Shed those pounds and quite likely your blood pressure will decrease, too.

Results of the Framingham project predict that each 10 percent reduction in weight reduces the risk of heart disease by 20 percent. Part of this reduction in risk is due to blood-pressure normalization (Ashley and Kannel, *British Medical Journal,* 1974). Perhaps Chapter 26 will help you to reduce. This may be all you need to return to good health free of the worry of premature death, kidney failure, or blindness.

Consider a Potassium Salt Substitute

Next, throw away your salt shaker or better, replace the salt with a potassium salt substitute (potassium chloride). Salt (sodium chloride) causes the body to retain water which, in turn, causes tissue swelling and increased blood volume. Tissue swelling means the heart has to pump harder in order to drive the pressure high enough to force the blood through the swollen tissue. Increased blood volume results in more fluid squeezing against the artery walls, thus your blood pressure is again increased. Vitamin C helps reduce the excess water retention, and potassium helps displace both the excess salt and water.

Not everyone experiences a rise in blood pressure with a rise in salt intake, but many do. The Africans, virtually free of heart disease, eat almost no salt and rarely get high blood pressure. In northern Japan, people eat about 30 grams of salt daily with the result that half of them die of stroke, a frequent complication of high blood pressure (N. Sasaki, *Geriatrics,* 1964). On the other hand, Buddhist farmers in Thailand with an average salt consumption of 20 grams daily have normal blood pressure even in old age.

Americans are great snack-food eaters, and food processors have learned that high levels of finely ground salt keep us reaching for the potato chips and pretzels. We eat about 10 to 20 grams of salt every day on the average, yet we need only 4 grams a day. Reduce your salt intake and talk to your doctor about using a salt substitute.

Selenium or Vitamin E Can Lower Your Blood Pressure

Selenium is an essential nutrient in the control of high blood pressure. Dr. J. E. Vincent (of Rotterdam Medical School, Erasmus University) has demonstrated that selenium is required for the production of certain prostaglandins (*Prostaglandins,* 1974).

Prostaglandin A₂, manufacturered in the kidney medulla, controls blood pressure. Hours after Dr. James B. Lee (of the Department of Medicine, State University of New York at Buffalo) infused prostaglandin A₂ into patients with high blood pressure, they experienced a normalization of blood pressure (*Laboratory Management,* 1974). Dr. Lee has also observed that the level of prostaglandin A₂ is much lower than normal in those patients with high blood pressure Some of the deficiency may be genetically caused and some may result from a dietary deficiency of selenium. It is reasonable to expect 100 micrograms of selenium added to the diet daily would be beneficial for those with high blood pressure. Selenium-rich foods include eggs, tuna, grains, garlic, and onions.

Vitamin E also normalizes blood pressure in many individuals. Vitamin E spares selenium in many body functions, thus freeing selenium for prostaglandin A₂ production. Additionally, vitamin E blocks the production of other prostaglandins (some of which may serve to constrict blood vessels), thus reducing their ability to elevate the blood pressure.

The roles of vitamin C, vitamin B₁₅, potassium, lecithin, and garlic in lowering blood pressure have already been discussed in earlier chapters, which you may wish to reread.

Don't forget that excess sugar can elevate the blood pressure (Ahrens, 1974), and that it hinders our ability to deal with stress (Cheraskin, 1974).

Biofeedback—It's Mind Over Matter

Stress has long been associated with increasing blood pressure—which is one of the body's reactions to stress stimuli. When danger threatens, the heart beats faster, and the pressure increases to feed the large muscles that may be called into action to protect the individual against the threat of danger. Unfortunately, today's stress is not usually a sudden danger, but a prolonged worry. The body reacts the same way, increasing blood pressure in the process. The control of stress is discussed in Chapter 29, but it should be noted here that, with the assistance of your sphygmomanometer, you can learn to control your body to lower your blood pressure. What you do is develop thoughts or feelings that calm you and lower your blood pressure slightly.

Biofeedback is the technique of training yourself to recognize and control physiological functions such as blood pressure, pulse, and brainwaves. Transcendental Meditation (TM) is a process of quieting mental activity completely spontaneously, with no manipulative learning process. With the practice of either technique you can develop a relaxation response that will produce greater drops in pressure. You may, like some people, develop the ability to completely master blood-pressure control. It's mind over matter, TM, and anything else you want to call it; but this form of biofeedback does work. Even elementary breathing exercises are helpful. Refer to Chapter 29 for more information on these procedures. And, especially, don't forget to cut your smoking.

Drugs—Some Are Far Safer Than Others

There are more than 50 drugs to lower blood pressure. Table 23.1 lists those most widely prescribed. Some will work for some people, but not others. Because the causes of high blood pressure are not fully understood, the drugs take a shotgun approach toward working on entire systems. Some widely used drugs are very harmful, resulting in drowsiness, dizziness, sexual impotence, or cancer. Often patients quit their medication because they feel all right with high blood pressure, but feel awful when taking medicine to lower it. If you are on medication, be sure to use the dietary cures to lower the dosages of medicine you require. Help your physician find the best drug for you. Whichever dietary cure you use, stick with it if it works. Whatever you do, normalize your blood pressure.

Historically, it has been believed that primary high blood

Table 23.1

Widely Prescribed Drugs for High Blood Pressure

Product	Brand	Mfr.	Dosage
Bendroflumethiazide	Naturetin	Squibb	5 mg tab
Bendroflumethiazide & rauwolfia serpentina	Rauzide	Squibb	Tab
Chlorthalidone & reserpine	Regroton	USV	Tab
Chlorothiazide & reserpine	Diupres	MS&D	250 mg tab
			500 mg tab
Clonidine HCl	Catapres	Boehringer	0.1 mg tab
			0.2 mg tab
Clonidine HCl & chlorthalidone	Combipres	Boehringer	0.1 mg tab
			0.2 mg tab
Guanethidine sulfate	Ismelin	Ciba	10 mg tab
			25 mg tab
Guanethidine monosulfate & hydrochlorthizide	Esimil	Ciba	Tab
Hydralazine HCl	Apresoline	Ciba	25 mg tab
			50 mg tab
Hydralazine HCl & hydrochlorothiazide	Apresoline Esidrix	Ciba	Tab
Hydralazine HCl, Hydrochlorothiazide & reserpine	Ser-ap-es	Ciba	Tab
Hydrochlorothiazide & reserpine	Hydropres	MS&D	50 mg tab
Hydrochlorothiazide & reserpine	Serpasil Esidrix	Ciba	No. 1 tab
			No. 2 tab

Product	Brand	Mfr.	Dosage
Methyclothiazide & cryptenamine tennates	Diutensen	Mallinckrodt	Tab
Methyclothiazide, crypetenamine tannates & reserpine	Diutensen-R	Mallinckrodt	Tab
Methychlothiazide & deserpidine	Enduronyl	Abbott	Tab
Methychlothiazide & deserpidine	Enduronyl Forte	Abbott	Tab
Methyldopa	Aldomet	MS&D	250 mg tab
			500 mg tab
Methyldopa & hydrochlorothiazide	Aldoclor-250	MS&D	Tab
Methyldopa & hydrochlorothiazide	Aldoril, Merseals 25	MS&D	
Metolazone	Zaroxolyn	Pennwalt	2.5 mg tab
			5 mg tab
Pargyline HCl	Eutron	Abbott	Tab
Polythiazide & reserpine	Renese R	Pfizer	Tab
Rauwolfia serpentina	Raudixin	Squibb	100 mg tab
Rauwolfia serpentina, bendroflumethiazide & potassium CL	Rautrax-N	Squibb	Tab
Reserpine	Serpasil	Ciba	.25 mg tab
Reserpine, hydrochlorothiazide	Butiserpazide	McNeil	25 mg tab
			50 mg tab

List is attributed to Medical Services Administration, Social & Rehabilitation Service, DHEW.

pressure is due to an abnormality either in the automatic nervous system or in certain glandular systems. Drugs that affect these systems can effectively lower the blood pressure, but most doctors feel this approach is like using a shotgun when only a bullet would be needed if they knew specifically where to aim. In other words, present drugs probably lower the blood pressure without getting at the specific mechanism that triggers it. Often several drugs have to be used, which sometimes produces dangerous side effects.

Several researchers are investigating the possibility that primary high blood pressure may be caused by a metabolic defect in the smooth muscle of blood-vessel walls (Samir Amer and Gordon McKinney, 58th Annual Meeting of the Federation of American Societies for Experimental Biology, 1974.) The overproduction of the kidney enzyme angiotensin, or the underproduction of the enzyme kallikrein are also being tested as possible causes of high blood pressure. When the cause of high blood pressure is more clearly identified, research will hopefully be able to develop a specific drug with fewer side effects.

The available drugs for primary high blood pressure fall roughly into four classes of compounds: adrenoceptor antagonists, peripherally acting compounds, centrally acting compounds, and diuretics. Often combinations of these main classes of antihypertensive drugs are used. (Additional classes of drugs are available for secondary hypertension.)

- *Adrenoceptor antagonists* block or inhibit the action of the hormone noradrenaline, a chemical messenger that carries sympathetic nerve impulses (those not initiated by conscious thought) to the various organs—particularly the heart and blood vessels.
- *Peripherally acting drugs* work by relaxing the muscle walls of blood vessels and increasing the extent of their dilation to reduce blood-vessel constriction.
- *Centrally acting drugs* affect the vasomotor center of the lower brain, which regulates the blood pressure.

- *Diuretics* remove water and salt, thus reducing both the blood volume and tissue pressure from edema.

Examples of adrenoceptor antagonists are guanethidine, reserpine (extracted from the Indian plant *Rauwolfia serpentina*), and compounds of the propanolamine class (as in the brand Inderal).

In September 1974, the Food and Drug Administration warned physicians through direct letters and press releases that women treated for high blood pressure with drugs containing reserpine may run a risk of breast cancer two to three times higher than those who have not taken the medicine. The warning was based on a collaborative study by researchers in Britain, Finland, and the United States (*Lancet,* 1974). The report, as explained by the senior U.S. investigator in the study (Dr. Herschel Jick of Boston), did not show cause and effect, because it was a retrospective study, but nevertheless it did indicate an association between reserpine and breast cancer.

Dr. Bruce Armstrong of Oxford University in England pointed out that the collaborative study confirmed an earlier 1972 study at Boston University Medical Center. Both studies showed the association only in women over 50 years of age. Reserpine, methoserpidine, deserpidine, and related drugs represent about 25 percent of the drugs used to treat high blood pressure in the United States.

Peripherally acting drugs include hydralazine (as in Apresoline) and dimethosyquinazolines (as in Prazosin). Diazoxide and nitroprusside also belong to this class, but are used only in emergencies. Occasionally, peripherally acting drugs increase salt retention; thus, diuretics are often used concurrently.

An example of the centrally acting drugs is clonidine (which occurs in Catapres). Tranquilizers such as Valium are often used alone or in combination with other drugs. Problems arising from centrally acting drugs are drowsiness, dizziness, and impotence.

The drugs guanethidine, methyldopa, bethanidine, clonidine, and spironolactone have been specifically indicated as causing sexual disorders (R. J. Newman, *British Medical Journal*, 1973 and 1975; E. Weil, *New England Journal of Medicine*, 1975). According to the reports, some drugs caused sexual problems in 50–70 percent of the men taking them. These drugs were bethanidine (with 67% of the male patients experiencing problems), methyldopa (affecting 60%) and quanethidine (affecting 54%). Symptoms include failure to sustain erection, failure to ejaculate, impotence, fatigue, lassitude, and inability to concentrate.

Milder side effects of several antihypertensive drugs include weakness, palpitation, constipation, dry mouth, sweating, nausea, vomiting, headache, insomnia, increased appetite, rash, nightmares, twitching, and hyperexcitability. If such side effects occur, your doctor should reduce your dosage or suggest another drug.

Diuretics include aldactone, thiazides, furosemide, ethacrynic acid, and chlorthalidone. Diuretics cause an increased production of urine to remove water and salt, but they also result in the increased excretion of all electrolytes, especially potassium. Patients taking diuretics must be sure to increase their consumption of high-potassium foods such as rice bran, wheat bran, sunflower seeds, wheat germ, almonds, parsley, sesame seeds, bananas, prunes, prune juice, tomatoes, tomato juice, raisins, and orange juice, or take potassium supplements, under their doctor's supervision. (For an understanding of the importance of potassium, see Chapter 15.) If you must take potassium, use the preferred forms described in that chapter. Some diuretics, such as triamterene or spironolactone, are potassium-sparing drugs.

Two diuretics have been shown to cause cancer in rats. The Food and Drug Administration warned physicians in January 1976 of the possible cancer risk of these drugs and discouraged physicians from prescribing aldactone and aldactazide—except when there are high blood levels of the hormone aldosterone, adrenal gland tumors, low potassium levels, or if all other methods have failed. The 78-week study of the drugs in rats was performed by the FDA.

Do not take enteric-coated formulations containing potassium. The enteric formulations (that will not dissolve until they reach the intestine) have caused small-bowel lesions, obstructions, hemorrhage, perforation, and death.

If your medication is among those mentioned above as dangerous, discuss alternative drugs with your doctor.

The Silent Enemy

High blood pressure is a common "silent" health problem that shortens life expectancy. The younger you are when you get high blood pressure, the more it will reduce your life expectancy.

By reducing your high blood pressure with diet, exercise, or drugs, you will reduce the risks of becoming a victim of stroke, heart failure, or kidney failure. (Remember most people with high blood pressure are unaware that they have it, because they feel well.)

High blood pressure requires constant attention. Once blood pressure is reduced to normal, treatment must be maintained or pressure will increase again. A person with high blood pressure can and should exercise as much as anyone else. If high blood pressure affected exercise, you would know it. Simple high blood pressure has few symptoms and is thought of as the "silent" killer. Normally it doesn't prevent you from exercising by causing discomfort. Complications of high blood pressure can cause heart damage. Heart damage—if caused by high blood pressure—is different. You know it, usually, and it limits your exercise.

Dietary control is important because weight reduction, salt and sugar restriction, plus vitamin and mineral supplementation, are all effective in normalizing blood pressure.

If your doctor has prescribed medication for your high blood pressure, you should take it exactly as instructed, even though you feel well. If you should feel ill, check with your doctor. Don't skip doses. Don't drop out of the treatment program.

Continue to check your blood pressure. (Figure 23.1 pro-

Figure 23.1

Blood Pressure Record
(For use by those with elevated blood pressure.)

Date	Time	Pressure	Pulse	Weight	Observations

vides a convenient and permanent record.) Be sure you don't get lulled into a false sense of security because you feel well. High blood pressure doesn't make you feel bad until damage is done. Stop or reduce smoking, learn to relax, and get daily exercise.

Smoking—The Grave Facts

Don't skip this chapter just because you don't smoke. Non smokers need protection too, because they breathe the nicotine and carcinogens from the smoke of others. Even those amounts can be enough exposure to warrant the full protection of Supernutrition. If you are a smoker, it's dangerous not to take vitamins C and E. And you can definitely use the extra protection of other nutrients. Smoking is the second most severe risk factor in heart disease (after high blood pressure).

Several studies, according to a 1964 American Heart Association booklet (EME 343 PHE), found "that death rates from heart attacks in men range from 50 to 200 percent higher among cigarette smokers than among non-smokers, depending on age and amount smoked. The average increase in [heart-attack] death rate [for smokers] is 70 percent."

An early report of the Framingham Study indicated that the risk of a heart attack or sudden death is three times as great for a male smoking 20 cigarettes daily as for a non-smoker (Doyle et al, *Journal of the American Medical Association,* 1964).

Men aged 25 who have never smoked can expect to average 6½ years of life more than men who smoke one pack or more a day (American Cancer Society booklet "If You Want to Give Up Cigarettes" 69-4R-250M-3/73 No. 2021).

A report by Dr. G. H. Miller (Assistant Director of Institutional Research at Edinboro State College in Pennsylvania) estimated that men who smoke two or more packs of cigarettes daily shorten their lives 14 to 15 years. The same amount of smoking among women cuts 19 to 20 years from their average lifespan (*Journal of Breathing,* 1975).

The Framingham study found that middle-aged men who smoke more than a pack of cigarettes a day are six times more likely to have strokes than middle-aged male non-smokers, regardless of any other risk factors.

In 1971, Britain's Royal College of Physicians reported, "Cigarette smoking is now as important a cause of death as were the great epidemic diseases such as typhoid, cholera and tuberculosis." They went on to estimate that deaths throughout the world caused by cigarettes in just one year exceed all the deaths from typhoid in Western Europe since the fifteenth century, all the TB epidemics in Europe since the eighteenth century, and all known epidemics of yellow fever in history.

Dr. C. Wilhemsson (of Sahlgren's Hospital of the University of Göteborg in Sweden) recommends that patients who survive a myocardial infarction (heart attack) should be strongly discouraged from smoking. Dr. Wilhemsson and his colleagues found that men who continue to smoke two years after their first infarction have twice the rate of rein-farction, cardiovascular deaths, and total mortality of men who have stopped smoking. Further, more smokers than nonsmokers die suddenly when an infarction occurs (*Lancet,* 1975).

A report on the Framingham data by Drs. Philip A. Wolf, Thomas R. Dawber, and Patricia M. McNamara (of the Boston University Medical Center) and Dr. William B. Kannel (of the National Institutes of Health) emphasized that "among men, the impact of cigarette smoking is strongest and significant in the ages 45 to 54. This effect wanes with increasing age. . . ."

Dr. Carl C. Seltzer of the Harvard School of Public Health in Boston observed that cigarette smoking after the age of 65 will not increase the risks of a heart attack.

If you are one of the smokers who lives through your 40s and 50s without a heart attack, your genes have probably helped you. But what a gamble.

Cigarette Sales Are Again on the Increase

In 1967, New York State Commissioner of Health Dr. Hollis S. Ingraham described cigarettes as being "more lethal for Americans than all the bullets, germs, and viruses combined." (WNBC-TV program *Direct Line.*)

Yet, cigarette sales are breaking records as more young people start smoking. There are now 50 million smokers in the United States. There were 875,000 more smokers in the U.S. in 1975 than in 1970. But it's not just the number of smokers and total quantity of cigarettes that's rising, it's the average number of cigarettes smoked per *person* (both smokers and nonsmokers) aged 18 and over. According to U.S. Dept. of Agriculture figures, the average dropped from the all-time high of 4,345 cigarettes a year in 1963 (just before the Surgeon General's Advisory Committee on Smoking and Health declared smoking was related to lung cancer and heart disease) to a low of 3,970 a year in 1970. Since then, the average (for smokers and nonsmokers) increased to 4,042 in 1971 and 4,050 in 1972.

The biggest increase (100 percent) in smoking habits has occurred among girls aged 12 to 17. Previously, a large increase in smoking had occurred among adult women. In 1965, 52.4 percent of American men over 21 were smokers; this dropped to 42.2 percent in 1970 and 39.3 percent in 1975. Among adult women, the percentage smoking was 32.5 percent in 1965, 42.2 percent in 1970, and 28.9 percent in 1975.

A smoker consuming just one pack a day will ingest almost 10 grams of nicotine and 125 grams of tar each year. The nicotine from 5 cigarettes can kill a rabbit; the nicotine from 100 cigarettes can kill a horse. Nicotine is highly toxic to man as well. It is one of the most powerful poisons, acting with the rapidity of cyanide. One-tenth of a drop (1/50 gram) can cause severe poisoning in humans. The tar causes cancer and monoclonal proliferation, but we have no toxicity numbers yet.

The Federal Trade Commission hopes to change the printed warning on cigarette packs and in cigarette ads from "Warning: The Surgeon General Has Determined That Cigarette Smoking Is Dangerous to Your Health" to "Warning: Cigarette Smoking Is Dangerous to Health and May Cause Death from Cancer, Coronary Heart Disease, Chronic Bronchitis, Pulmonary Emphysema and Other Diseases." They have an alternate choice in "Warning: Cigarette Smoking Is a Major Health Hazard and May Result in Your Death."

How Smoking Endangers Your Health

Smoking affects heart health in many ways, but the biggest problem it causes is the increased tendency of the blood to form clots. In addition, reports that nicotine decreases the body's ability to dissolve blood clots have appeared in the scientific literature.

Dr. Rosemary Hawkins of the Huntington Research Centre in England found that smokers experienced increased platelet aggregation. (See Chapter 9.) In the occasional smoker, some of the changes occurred only immediately after smoking, but in heavy smokers the changes persisted even through periods of nonsmoking (*Nature,* 1972).

Dr. Peter H. Levine of Tufts School of Medicine in Boston has found that inhaling the smoke of even one cigarette quickly increases the platelet adhesion in humans.

Thus, smoking a cigarette can trigger a fatal blood clot in someone already having narrowed arteries, poor circulation, and a high platelet-adhesion index.

Smoking just one cigarette can cause other severe effects in the circulation system. Dr. Po-Cheng Chang of the University of Utah reports that smoking one cigarette constricted peripheral vascular lumen size (arterial opening space) in humans to one-quarter its normal area, nearly doubling the artery-wall thickness and reducing the artery's elasticity by more than 50 percent.

Smoking just one cigarette also increases the pulse an extra 15 to 25 beats per minute, and the increase may persist up to 20 minutes after the last puff. For the average smoker, that's more than 10,000 extra beats a day for your heart. At the same time blood pressure is increased by 10 to 20 points (mm/mercury) because nicotine constricts the blood vessels—especially those of the extremities. The poor circulation caused by smoking can be detected by a thermograph (temperature-sensitive instrument), which often will indicate a temperature drop of 10° F or more in a smoker's hands and feet after just a few puffs. Dr. Phillip Cryer of the Washington University School of Medicine showed that the blood pressure increases within 5 minutes and that the hormone norepinephrine increases in the blood within 10 minutes (*New England Journal of Medicine,* 1976).

Nicotine is a powerful drug that, although socially acceptable and legally sanctioned, indirectly kills more citizens in the United States each year than heroin and car accidents combined.

Smoking Causes Oxygen Starvation

Besides being burdened with increased platelet adhesion, the blood of a smoker is less capable of doing its job of supplying oxygen to the body. Gases in the smoke (carbon monoxide and hydrogen cyanide—both deadly poisons) tie up the red blood cells, preventing them from carrying oxygen to the cells and slowing down their release of oxygen to the cells when they can transport oxygen.

Smoking also destroys or congests the lung's alveoli, the air sacs in which the exchange of carbon dioxide in the blood for oxygen takes place.

All smokers know that their "wind" is affected by their smoking. This occurs when muscle action slows because of insufficient oxygen. Smokers should realize that this reserve they miss in muscle action is the same reserve that could save their life if the blood to their heart were reduced by a clot in one of the coronary arteries. If enough oxygen still gets through to the heart, it survives and you can live a normal life when it heals.

Smoking Can Cause Deposits in the Arteries

In addition to the fact that smoking causes clots and oxygen starvation, there is still another major problem. Smoking can start the process of plaque deposits in the artery.

Cigarette smoke contains benzopyrene, which can trigger the monoclonal cell proliferation itself. And other smoke components cause reactions in the blood that produce mal-aldehyde, another compound that triggers cell proliferation.

Smoking is not the only source of free radicals and mutagenic compounds, but if you smoke, you are constantly exposing your body to considerable quantities of these deleterious chemicals, and eventually they may overcome your body's defense mechanism.

Cigarette Smoke Is High in Harmful Cadmium

Tobacco smoke also contains cadmium, which besides being a toxic metal, raises the blood pressure. More cadmium can enter the body from cigarette smoke (1.5 micrograms per pack) than from the diet and drinking water (less than 1 microgram daily). The more cigarettes smoked, the more cadmium is stored in vital organs, eventually leading to high blood pressure.

For Women—You've Come a Long Way, Baby, but It's Costing You 20 Years

The increased smoking rate among women is having a disastrous effect on their death rate. Female smokers were found to die at an average age of 59, compared to 65 for male smokers, according to the report by Dr. Miller mentioned at the beginning of this chapter. His study found nonsmokers, both men and women, lived to an average of 75 to 76 years in the 4,000 deaths studied.

Other investigators have found similar results. During the 1950s in Westchester County, N.Y., there were twelve coronary deaths for men to every one for women. During 1967 to 1972, the ratio fell to four to one (*Journal of the American Medical Association,* 1973).

The researchers (Dr. David M. Spain at Brookdale Hospital in Brooklyn and Drs. Henry Siegel and Victoria A. Bradess of the Westchester County Medical Examiners Office) concluded that the reason women are rapidly approaching the heart-disease death rate of men is an increase in heavy smoking. They predict the trend will worsen, as did Dr. Miller.

In the Westchester County Study of those succumbing from heart attacks, the women who smoked a pack or more of cigarettes daily died at an average age of 19 years younger than women who were nonsmokers. (The non-smoking women who died of heart disease averaged 67 years of age, whereas the smoking women who died of heart disease averaged 48 years of age.)

Heart disease is twice as prevalent among women smoking ten or more cigarettes daily than among women non-smokers aged 45 to 54, according to Dr. Daniel Horn, Director of the National Clearinghouse for Smoking and Health.

The heart-disease death rate for women is increasing dramatically. Women are under a double-barreled attack from the dangers of smoking and "the pill." Both cigarette smoke and the birth-control pill significantly increase the blood-platelet adhesion index.

If you smoke *or* take "the pill," you should, in my opinion, also take vitamin E. If you smoke and take "the pill," you may find alternate contraceptive techniques healthier. If you prefer the pill to other methods, you are best advised to discontinue smoking.

Nonsmokers Are Damaged by Others' Smoke

If you work or live with smokers, you are a "passive smoker." Smokers generally don't realize how much cigarette smoke irritates the throat, eyes, and lungs of nonsmokers, because smokers lose their tissue sensitivity through constant exposure. Even nonsmokers are unaware of the amounts of nicotine that can be picked up just by being in the same room as a smoker.

Dr. M. A. H. Russel (at Maudsley Hospital, London) and Dr. C. Feyerabend (at New Cross Hospital, London) found that most nonsmokers have measurable amounts of nicotine in their body fluids (and the only source of nicotine is tobacco).

A study at Texas A & M University by Drs. Carl W. Landers and Donald J. Marki proved that smoke in a poorly ventilated room significantly increases the heart rate, blood pressure, and carbon monoxide level of the blood of nonsmokers.

Even cadmium from other peoples' cigarettes can pollute your body. In 1971, Dr. H. G. Petering, Environmental Health Professor at the University of Cincinnati, reported at a meeting of the American Chemical Society that 6 percent of the cadmium in a cigarette is inhaled by the smoker, but 50 percent goes into the surrounding air (the rest, 44 percent, remains in the ash). Dr. Petering found that in a 10' × 12' room, the smoking of just one pack of cigarettes over an eight-hour period increased the cadmium in the air more than 10 times above normal. And remember, cadmium increases blood pressure.

The carbon monoxide from cigarette smoke ties up the hemoglobin of the red blood cells, thus reducing the oxygen-carrying capability of the blood. This can be serious to people with angina, atherosclerosis, or myocardial infarction. Yet your lungs and blood can get high levels of carbon monoxide from the smokers around you, even if you've never smoked in your life.

Dr. Raymond C. Slavin of St. Louis University observed that just sitting in a room with smokers quadrupled the carbon monoxide level (10 parts per million) in a nonsmoker's lungs, enough to cause a headache and a dull, tired feeling in otherwise healthy people.

To this pollution from smokers, add the carbon monoxide pollution from auto exhausts and you can see that even nonsmokers must actively protect themselves from passive pollutants that can damage their hearts.

Protection for Smokers and Nonsmokers

As can be seen from the preceding discussions, giving up smoking is an important step in preventing heart disease, but that alone is not enough, because the smoke from others' cigarettes can damage your heart. Therefore, you must help your body defend itself against the unnatural biological insult from the ingredients of tobacco smoke that man was not designed to handle.

The first priority is to normalize the blood-platelet adhesion index. Vitamin E can do that. It can also increase the oxygen-carrying ability of the blood and reduce the membrane damage that can lead to plaque formation in the arteries.

As a rule of thumb, nonsmokers are generally protected by 400 to 800 IU daily, while smokers receive protection from 800 to 1,600 IU, depending on how heavily they smoke. (Diabetics and those on heart medications should read pages 106 to 110 to review the precautions they must observe when initiating a vitamin E program.) Even a pound of vitamin E can't bring full protection to a heavy smoker, but some protection is better than none.

The cadmium in smoke can be partially tied up and thus detoxified by selenium. The supplemental needs for selenium vary according to the amount in the foods you eat. Smokers should consider taking 50 to 150 micrograms daily in supplements. (See Chapter 32 for details.)

Vitamin B_{15} has helped many smokers, especially those with emphysema. I have received many letters from people explaining the relief they obtained with vitamin B_{15} (which spares oxygen by detoxifying oxygen-consuming impurities and increases tissue respiration). B_{15} has brought about seemingly miraculous cures of heart disease, especially angina.

Harald Taub, past editor of *Let's LIVE* magazine, remarked in an April 1976 editorial: "Like every heavy smoker, I have long suffered from the symptoms of oxygen insufficiency. I quickly become short of breath on exercising. If I take a long walk, I get pains in my legs. When the weather becomes quite damp, I have trouble catching my breath. Or, at least all these things were true for many years. They began improving about two weeks after I started taking a supplement of vitamin B$_{15}$. I have continued to take the supplement and the improvement has been steady.

"I no longer breathe heavily when I'm sitting at my desk. I no longer wake up in the middle of a foggy night gasping for breath. I am once again able to walk almost without limit without any discomfort. I am convinced that these improvements have come about as a result of adding vitamin B$_{15}$ to the other good nutrients that I had already been taking, and I am eager to go on taking vitamin B$_{15}$ for the rest of my life."

How much do you need? That depends on you and your lifestyle, but heavy smokers should consider 150 milligrams daily.

Measurements of vitamin C levels in smokers' blood have been low enough to indicate that smokers should take at least 25 milligrams of vitamin C for each cigarette smoked (or 500 mg for each pack) just to compensate for the loss. This is, of course, in addition to your daily need for vitamin C, which may be 2 or 3 grams or more. Review Chapter 14 for details on the relationship between vitamin C deficiency and heart disease.

Those subjected to tobacco smoke also need adequate intakes of vitamin A. Some components of cigarette smoke destroy vitamin A on the spot. Therefore, some of the vitamin A that's in your foods is wasted by the smoke in your lungs. You need extra vitamin A to maintain the health of your lungs as well as to protect against monoclonal proliferation.

Smokers should be especially aware that vitamin A has been shown to protect against spontaneous, chemically caused, and transplanted cancers (Bjelke, *International Journal of Cancer,* 1975; Hill and Shih, *Cancer Research,* 1974; also *Science,* December 1974; *American Journal of Clinical Nutrition,* 1973; and Saffioti, Ninth International Cancer Congress, October 1966).

Again the optimum amount of any vitamin varies from person to person, but 20,000 to 35,000 IU seem to be best for most people. The heavy smoker could use 10,000 IU additionally.

Other nutrients that are especially important if you smoke are zinc, manganese, pectin, lecithin, sulfur-containing amino acids such as cysteine, and seaweed alginate.

Smokers Need More Exercise

A safety measure for smokers is exercise. Dr. C. M. Frank pointed out that an inactive smoker is twice as likely to die from his first heart attack as an active smoker, and nine times as likely to die from his first heart attack as an active nonsmoker (*Journal of American Medical Association* 1966).

The more active you are, the better your chances, whether you smoke or not, and that says a lot for exercising. Chapter 25 discusses exercising and its benefits and Chapter 26 describes a few good exercises to get you going.

25
Kicking the Smoking Habit

Protecting yourself against cigarette smoke with nutrients is very important, but the full protection is possible only when you kick the habit. There is strong evidence that after a few years of abstinence, the former smoker's risk of heart attack becomes nearly the same as that of a nonsmoker of the same age. The biggest factor in breaking the smoking habit is wanting to. When you decide you want to stop smoking, you can. Thirty million former smokers have.

Choose a method of quitting that best suits your personality. Some do better by stopping all at once; others are more comfortable gradually reducing the number of cigarettes smoked each day, and still others are able to quit by picking a target date on which they will stop.

Choose a system that doesn't scare you or offend you. But, even before that, determine why you smoke. Is it to reduce stress? To relax? To feel accepted? Because of hypoglycemia (low blood sugar)? Habit? Craving? Stimulation? Or to have something in your hands? Once you identify the main reason why you smoke, then you can select a program for that particular problem.

Methods To Help You Stop

A "craver" can spoil his craving for cigarettes by smoking too much for a couple of days and then stopping. A "stresser" does better by trying to stop during a lax period or vacation—never under stress. A "handler" can get along by just handling the cigarette and never lighting it. A "stimulator'' can be satisfied with large amounts of B vitamins or by chewing on a ginger root or clove. The "habitual" smoker should try a mouthwash after meals, rather than a cigarette.

The "wrapper method" is helpful for those who want to cut down over a period of time. A sheet of ruled standard notebook paper is wrapped around the pack of cigarettes and secured with two or three rubber bands. Everytime you get an urge to smoke, unwrap the package and record the day, date, time, cigarette and pack number, what you are doing (activity), how you feel, the importance to you of that cigarette, a reason to stop smoking and whether or not you decide to smoke that cigarette. At the end of the day, study the list to see how many cigarettes you smoked merely out of habit, because someone else offered one, to go along with your coffee, etc. The "casual" cigarette can often be avoided if you simply become aware of it. And that's a good start right there. Later, when you start discarding the "important" ones, the process will be easier than it would have been, because you'll be giving up up fewer cigarettes at the "breakpoint."

A variation of the wrapper method is to close the pack with transparent tape. You can carry the pack, but getting to the cigarette is more difficult, and the urge to smoke may leave before the pack can be opened.

Some people have done better by taping pictures of loved ones on the pack. Thus, when they see the picture, they receive pleasant thoughts that dispel the need for the cigarette, or they strengthen their determination to quit for the benefit of the loved ones. In other smokers, this method causes a feeling of guilt which is undesirable. You shouldn't quit because you feel guilty, and you probably won't. So, if a method causes guilt, try another. Quitting should be a relaxed process with no pressure from anyone.

Helpful tricks include putting the money for a week's worth of cigarettes in an envelope, and opening it to buy only one pack of cigarettes at a time. The money not spent can be taped to a large calendar as a graphic demonstration of money saved and progress towards a goal.

The craving for nicotine goes away in about a week, but

even during the week, the craving hits only occasionally and lasts only for ten minutes at a time. Look at your watch when it hits, and realize that in ten minutes the craving will leave —whether you smoke or not.

Remember that alcohol will increase the nicotine craving and lessen your will power.

Giving up smoking will be one of the major events of your life. You'll feel like a hero when you've done it. You'll be setting an example for your family and friends. You may help save their lives, as well as your own.

Deep Breathing May Help

If you smoke to relax, you will find it easy to replace cigarettes with a relaxing substitute, such as eating fruit, drinking water, chewing gum, or deep breathing.

Deep-breathing methods have helped many, and the techniques vary from simple to complicated. The simplest is, when you get a desire to smoke, to just take a deep breath and hold it as long as you can without great discomfort, then exhale and breathe normally. This procedure gives you a pause from your activity, breaks the tension, gives you something to do, a chance to decide if you really need the cigarette, and a pleasant feeling when the uncomfortable feeling of holding your breath is relieved. It also gives you a challenge—to see if you can hold your breath longer each day.

A more complicated deep-breathing technique claims an 80 percent success rate in helping people stop smoking. It was developed by William P. Knowles in England. Three times a day the following five steps are repeated:

1) Sit erect in a chair without allowing your back to rest against the chair.
2) Stretch your arms forward as far as you can without moving your back. Then slowly pull them back towards your chest by bending your elbows. Let your palms rest on your thighs and your elbows rest against the sides of your body.

3) Quickly and forcibly inhale and exhale through your nose twelve times.
4) Exhale slowly and completely, driving out all of the air that you can force out.
5) Inhale deeply during seven counts. Hold the air in for one full second, then exhale completely.

Do seven cycles of steps 3, 4, and 5 (complete exhales and inhales). That's all there is to it.

The Nuisance Principle

Another technique works on the nuisance principle and takes the enjoyment out of smoking, if that's the reason you smoke. Dr. Johannes Brengelman at Munich's Max Planck Institute designed this method with 11 steps.

1) Decide that you will smoke one, two, or three fewer cigarettes each day.
2) Change your cigarette brand with every pack.
3) After your first puff on a cigarette, put it out, then relight it and finish it.
4) Put your cigarette in the ashtray after every puff. Don't hold it in your hands.
5) Clean your ashtray after every cigarette.
6) If you are watching TV, turn it off during the time you smoke.
7) Don't smoke while you read or read while you smoke.
8) Don't smoke and eat or drink at the same time.
9) Don't leave cigarettes in plain view.
10) Don't carry cigarettes with you. Keep them in a drawer.
11) Keep your matches or lighter in a different room than your cigarettes—or at least in a different part of the room.

Whichever method you choose can be helped by drinking massive amounts of water and juices to flush out nicotine. Try warm baths just before bed and cool showers to start the day. Take walks after every meal, followed by relaxing, deep breathing. In enclosed public places sit in "no smoking" areas.

Commercial Aids

Some people are helped by the various aids you buy, others find them of no use. Scientific studies have produced mixed results. Some studies show that lobeline sulfate (Bantron), a nicotine substitute, helps four out of five, while other tests show nearly the same effectiveness for sugar pills when the smokers were told the pills were an effective drug to help stop smoking.

Similar findings have resulted from the temporary use of tranquilizers, sedatives, stimulants, and nicotine itself, in the form of chewing gum or tablets. The method that works for you is mostly a matter of your personality. The same goes for cigarette holders that gradually taper you off by diluting the smoke with air, audio tapes that reinforce the suggestion that you won't smoke, or flavored candies or mints that turn terrible tasting in your mouth when you smoke.

Groups to Help You Give Up Smoking

Most smokers can break the habit themselves; others do better in groups sharing common problems. Where can you get more details? Write or call any of the following:

- American Cancer Society
    219 East 42nd St.
    New York, N.Y. 10017
    (or local chapter)
- American Heart Association
    44 East 23rd St.
    New York, N.Y. 10010
    (or local chapter)

- Interagency Council on Smoking and Health
  (a joint organization of the ACS and AHA, with several local chapters)
- Mind Control and Meditation
  (check classified ads and yellow pages for TM and other centers)
- National Clearinghouse for Smoking and Health
  5401 Westbard Avenue
  Bethesda, Md. 20016
- National Tuberculosis and Respiratory Disease Association
  1740 Broadway
  New York, N.Y. 10019
- Shick Center to Control Smoking
  (local chapters, or call Los Angeles Headquarters, 215–553–9771)
- Seventh-Day Adventists
  c/o Dorcas Welfare Society
  6840 Eastern Ave., N.W.
  Washington, D. C. 20012
  (or contact local church)
- SmokEnders
  Parkway Office Bldg.
  Phillipsburg, N. J. 08865
- Smoke Watchers
  185 Fifth Ave.
  New York, N.Y. 10020
  (or local clinic)

Withdrawal Symptoms and How to Handle Them

It won't be easy at first, or you would have quit smoking long ago. But don't become discouraged at the first sign of a withdrawal symptom.

An expert in helping people kick the smoking habit, Dr. Arthur Weaver of Wayne State University in Detroit, offers the following suggestions for handling the withdrawal symptoms:

1) Nervousness—Expect it and allow for it. Warn your friends. It will disappear in a few days. Don't worry, you won't be nervous the rest of your life.
2) Lethargy—Some ex-smokers feel dull and depressed for a few days. (I suggest extra B vitamins.)
3) Restlessness—About 10 percent become restless or hyperactive. (I recommend taking warm baths at bedtime, and lining up some simple tasks to putter around with.)
4) Headache—An occasional person will develop headaches when the nicotine-constricted blood vessels return to normal size. This usually disappears by the third day, and aspirins will get you through.
5) Sore Throat—An occasional symptom, like headache. The nerves in the throat are returning to normal. Try cough drops. It will only last a day or two.
6) Breathlessness—Your imagination. When you stop smoking, breathing becomes easier, and you are not as aware of taking a breath.
7) About 8 percent of those kicking the habit have increased appetite, but that can be controlled after you have adjusted to your nonsmoking.

Weight Gain

People who stop smoking sometimes turn to overeating. Some substitute candy and snacks for cigarettes. Others say that food tastes better when they don't smoke. Perhaps the appetite mechanism has been suppressed by the nicotine. If you are not careful, you could gain up to 15 or 20 pounds when you kick the habit; but fortunately, most put on only 3 or 4 pounds.

A five-year study of 500 men sponsored by the National Heart, Lung, and Blood Institute determined that the average weight gain was 3.7 pounds. This small weight gain, even if not taken off, is healthier than smoking. Drs. George W. Cornstock and Richard W. Stone, the researchers of the weight-gain study, concluded the weight gain was subcutaneous (beneath-the-skin) fat, which is not necessarily associated with an increased risk of mortality. They also emphasized that there is a decreased mortality rate when smoking is discontinued.

Furthermore, another study has shown that quitting smoking does not cause weight gain in men over 45 years old. Drs. Raymond Bosse and Arthur Garvey of the Veterans Hospital in Boston found no link between quitting smoking and weight gain in males 45 years and older in a five-year study of 1,633 men over 45.

To minimize weight gain while kicking the habit, snack on celery, radishes, ginger, cucumbers, green peppers, carrots, lettuce, or bananas rather than candy.

Kicking the habit isn't easy, but 30 million smokers have quit. There are still 50 million smokers, because of population growth, but surveys show that 75 percent of them want to quit. When they really decide they would rather live in good health than smoke, they will be able to.

26
Calories Do Count

Obesity is serious. Fat on the belly means fat on the heart and fat-clogged arteries. Cholesterol doesn't count, but calories do.

It is harder for the heart to pump blood through the extra blood vessels required solely to nourish the fat. The increase in blood pressure means hypertension, with its accompanying heart damage. Fat people, as a result, are more subject to atherosclerosis.

The Metropolitan Insurance Company suggests that a person over 45 years of age who is a mere 10 pounds overweight decreases his lifespan by about 8 percent. For every additional 10 extra pounds, the person's risk of dying prematurely becomes 20 percent greater.

The American Heart Association predicts that your lifespan will be shortened (on the average) by 3.6 years if you are 25 percent overweight, 4.3 years if 35 percent overweight, 6.6 years at 45 percent overweight, and 11.4 years at 55 percent overweight.

Take a simple look at the basic mathematics of food calories and body weight. A pound of body fat averages 83 percent pure fat, with the rest being water and other materials stored in the fat. This pound of body fat would yield 3,500 calories when burned. When you eat 3,500 calories more than you burn, you will put on a pound of fat, regardless of whether it happens all in one day or over a year. Likewise, if you burn off 3,500 extra calories, you will lose a pound, whether in one day or one year.

Most people gain their fat slowly—1 or 2 pounds a year, generally beginning after the age of 25. By 45, people can be 25 to 50 pounds overweight, although they've only put on 1 or 2 pounds each year. It all starts with only 1 ½ to 2 ½ ounces a month, or a mere 10 or 20 extra calories a day—that's only one or two potato chips.

How Much Should You Weigh?

Body weight can be bone or muscle as well as fat. The weight tables are misleading, as they are for "average" people. You have a particular bone structure, and so much muscle. Are you overweight? The mirror will tell you. Do you paunch, sag, or hang? Can you grab a handful of flab on your stomach or your butt?

One guideline is not to exceed the body weight you had at age 25, unless you are now more muscular. If you're less muscular, subtract 5 pounds or so from your weight at 25. Needless to say, I am assuming that you were not fat at 25. If you were, here's one guideline you can forget.

How to Lose Weight

There are a few sane, practical ways of overcoming overweight that will work, but there are a thousand gimmicks touted that will not help . . . Eat all the food you want! Eat lots of your favorite foods! Wear this. Drink this. Hogwash!

The only way to lose fat permanently is to eat fewer calories than you use. This isn't to say that popular diets, such as low-carbohydrate diets, where you don't count calories but count carbohydrates, don't work. They do! But they probably are not ideal for permanent maintenance. Incidentally, you do reduce your calorie intake on those diets, even though you don't count calories. I have known more people to lose weight by Dr. Atkins's diet than by any other diet. The diet is O.K. for losing 10 to 20 pounds quickly (in 5 to 8 weeks), but then balanced nutrition should be resumed to maintain the weight loss or to lose more weight.

Bruce Randall, a former Mr. Universe, went from 203 to

401 pounds in 21 months. His body weight was mostly muscle, but also included about 10 percent fat. To obtain this weight, he drank 12 quarts of milk a day, ate 28 eggs for breakfast, a loaf of bread at each meal, and so on. He found that 401 pounds was totally impractical to carry. It was expensive to maintain; he needed two seats when he traveled, clothes had to be tailor-made. He reduced from 401 to 183, a loss of 218 pounds, in 8 months.

His method was to remove one unit of a type of food each day, while maintaining his vigorous exercise activity. One day, he would eat one egg less; another day, one less piece of toast; the next day, one glass of milk less. In this manner, his stomach shrank gradually and he didn't suffer hunger pains at all. His "slow" reduction was about 7 pounds per week, but his exercise program helped keep his skin from sagging.

You might use that method. Eat one less slice of toast a day for the first week. Eat one less helping of potato or spaghetti for the second week.

The only gimmick about dieting is not to look for a gim-

Table 26.1

Average Daily Calorie Needs As Estimated by the National Research Council

Age (yrs.)	Wt. (lbs.)	Ht. (in.)	Calories
Women			
15–18	119	65	2,100
19–22	128	65	2,000
23–50	128	65	2,000
51+	128	65	1,800
Men			
15–18	134	69	3,000
19–22	147	69	3,000
23–50	154	69	2,700
51+	154	69	2,400

mick. There are no secret formulas, no shortcuts—only common sense and consistency.

If you eat just 39 calories more than you need at each meal, you will gain a pound a month, 12 pounds a year, or 60 pounds in just 5 years. Thirty-nine calories—that's only 3 crackers or 4 potato chips.

Looking at it the other way, if you eat 39 calories fewer than you need to maintain your present weight, you will lose a pound a month, or 12 pounds a year. If you add just a small amount of exercise, such as walking an extra mile a day—10 blocks away and back again—you will lose an extra pound each 36 days, for a total of 10 more pounds each year. Putting both together, you can lose 22 pounds a year without much effort.

How Fast Should You Lose Weight?

Bruce Randall's 7-pound-per-week weight loss was faster than ideal for most people. Two pounds a week is enough; that's 104 pounds a year. Losing weight at a faster rate causes you to lose lean protein along with the fat.

Do not expect much weight loss in the first 7 to 10 days. If you go slow, you learn to live with the diet and can maintain good eating habits. There are no put-off cravings and no false security that if you do gain weight, you can take it off in a month. When you lose weight too fast, you become short-tempered and undernourished.

How Much Should You Cut from Your Diet?

Dr. Michael J. Mahoney (Professor of Clinical Psychology at Penn State University) recommends multiplying your body weight by two. This gives you the number of calories that you should cut down each day. By doing this, you will lose 10 percent of your body weight over a six-month period, which is just about ideal.

Dieting Aids

There are pills and injections you can get. My advice is to avoid them. They are not without side effects. This includes diuretics, thyroid extracts, amphetamines, and fat-mobilizing hormones.

There is one exception to this rule. Bran tablets or methyl cellulose tablets are beneficial and useful in dieting. Methyl cellulose is similar to paper or celery stalk, and simply expands in your stomach and intestine to give you a feeling of being full. The tablets are not digested and are not absorbed by the body, but they are beneficial because they increase your dietary fiber and bulk, which helps stimulate proper bile secretion, lowers blood cholesterol levels, and keeps food moving along in the intestine so that it doesn't putrefy to enhance bowel cancer.

Rather than take methyl cellulose pills, you may prefer to eat celery, apples, lettuce, bran, and other leafy or fibrous foods to give you natural bulk.

Helpful Dieting Hints

1) Keep a "food diary." Record everything you eat for a week. *Everything!* Snacks included. Decide which snacks are merely habit and can be dispensed with, and slowly cut them back.
2) Carry a picture of yourself at a better weight.
3) Weigh yourself nude daily, each morning before breakfast. Look at the trends, but don't worry about temporary increases due to occasional water retention or slight irregularity.
4) Drink more water. It fills your stomach, makes you more comfortable, and washes away the waste products of fat metabolism. Take your vitamin pills with water before meals to help fill you up.
5) Eat slowly, thoroughly chewing your food. This gives your hunger-control center time to adjust to your food intake.
6) If you can't eat leisurely, postpone your meal until you can.
7) Eat more fresh fruits for dessert.

8) Increase your physical activity and exercise.
9) When tempted to eat a snack, first imagine yourself as fat as the refrigerator. Then take a drink of water while imagining yourself at ideal weight.
10) Don't snack while watching TV.
11) Reduce your TV viewing time and replace that time with activity or exercise; take long walks.
12) Park farther from work or the market. Walk at least part of every ride; give up riding whenever possible.
13) Climb several floors of stairs, then take the elevator the rest of the way.
14) Eat meals restaurant style, with a single serving of each food on the plate, rather than family style, where extra food stays on the table for second helpings.
15) Eat an apple at breakfast, celery at lunch, and sliced raw carrots at dinner.
16) Sublimate your food cravings by indulging in other pleasures.
17) Don't eat sugar foods after 7:00 P.M. or before 10:00 A.M.
18) Don't sleep more than eight hours a day. Don't try to compensate for lost sleep by eating more snacks for energy.
19) Make breakfast your largest meal of the day.
20) Know the calorie content of foods. Low-calorie foods can fill your stomach, while high-calorie foods put weight on you, but still leave you hungry. Make every calorie count, and count every calorie.
21) Have realistic goals, and reward yourself as you reach each goal.
22) Realize that your progress won't be steady. You will have plateaus or "sticking points" where you will stay at the same weight for a week or two. Don't be discouraged or say "what's the use?" Persist. Soon the progress will continue.
23) If you cheat your nutrition, you won't lose only fat, but needed protein and muscle. You will become irritable and grouchy.
24) Cut back *slightly* on salt, sugar, and spices. Not making some food too tasty will help.
25) Prepare less food, put less on the plates, and use smaller plates.
26) Learn to enjoy that hungry feeling that occurs during the

first two to three days of dieting. It is telling you, "It's working!" It's telling you that fat is burning off.
27) Remember that the B-complex vitamins (especially B$_6$ and pantothenic acid) are required to burn up fat.

During the stress of dieting, the intestinal tract must be kept in a healthy condition by stimulating the growth of favorable bacteria as against toxic types. This is accomplished by taking acidophilus lactobacillus both morning and evening. Drug and health-food stores carry acidophilus in capsules or liquid form. Recently, acidophilus sweet milk has become available at grocery stores and supermarkets.

Bananas (or, when you can't store or carry them, banana powder) have the property of depressing appetite when eaten about 20 minutes before mealtime, or in between meals when hunger is discomforting. The sweetness is enough for this purpose, and the carbohydrates present, as well as the natural fat content of the bananas, are helpful in satisfying the appetite. Potassium is an important ingredient of bananas and this tends to prevent the hypoglycemia which makes people nervous, hungry, and weak.

Avoid Large Meals

Overeating, both in terms of long-range weight gain and short-range effects on the heart, is detrimental.

I believe people would do better on four or five mini-meals rather than one, two, or three larger meals, because the body can more easily handle a regular supply of small quantities of food. Also, smaller meals produce fewer harmful free radicals. Just one large meal can bring on a heart attack, as explained below.

1) Enlargement of the stomach stimulates the vagus nerve, which tends to depress the heart beat.
2) The blood vessels of the digestive tract become enlarged in order to absorb the digested food. When they enlarge, they fill with a greater than normal amount of blood, and the heart has to work harder to supply the blood.

3) The distended stomach presses on the diaphragm and makes it harder to breathe. It may even transmit some pressure to the heart, making it harder for the heart to beat.

A person who has a heart attack after having overeaten will undoubtedly vomit. If the gastric contents are inhaled, this can cause death, either immediately, due to hypoxia (lack of oxygen), or later, due to aspiration pneumonia, which has an extremely high fatality rate.

In addition, consider that a heavy meal also overloads the body's fat-transport mechanism, causing an abnormal distribution of fats in the blood. Some researchers feel this abnormal distribution of fats contributes to atherosclerosis.

Large meals also increase the possibility of a "café coronary," in which lodged food causes death by choking but is at first mistaken for a heart attack.

If you survive a large meal, then you will be faced with the deadly problem of surviving many large meals—obesity. The American Public Health Association estimates that between 60 and 80 million Americans are overweight—nearly one out of three.

Food is to be enjoyed, and eating should be a pleasant sensation. But if you overindulge, that pleasure becomes a dangerous act. If you don't eat any more than in previous years, but seem to gain weight, it's because your needs are not as great as they were when you were more active. Either participate in more activity or eat less. Preferably, you will become more active.

27

Exercise Strengthens the Heart

The body was meant to be used. If it isn't used and well-nourished, it deteriorates. You attain your best possible health when you combine regular exercise and proper rest with vitamin supplements and a balanced diet. Too little activity and exercise makes you sluggish and causes your vital organs to waste away.

Use It or Lose It!

A high level of general daily activity is essential to good health. Bending, stretching, standing, walking, and climbing do more than burn calories. They stimulate muscle repair, improve circulation, tone and stimulate our internal organs.

Systematic exercising adds even further advantages. It eases stress, chases depression, improves sex, sleep, and immunity, lowers blood cholesterol (if that is important to you), strengthens bones, helps you think better, and leaves you with a general feeling of well-being and alertness for 10 to 12 hours afterward.

Data from the American Cancer Society shows that the death rate of men between the ages of 45 and 65 who exercise regularly is four times lower than that of those who don't. Dr. Paul Metzer, Associate Medical Director for the Nationwide Insurance Company, says, "Just because you are past 40, don't think you are too old for regular exercise.

Ten minutes of exercise will double the blood level of norepinephrine, a hormone related to adrenalin, which boosts your spirits and destroys depression."

Standing on your feet two hours daily increases bone strength and reduces the chance of having blood clots. Standing exerts longitudinal compression on major bones. This stimulates bone maintenance and prevents the bones from wasting away. Standing also prevents the blood from accumulating in the legs. Sitting tends to restrict the return of blood to the heart, which encourages clot formation.

The Ireland-Boston Heart Study (mentioned in Chapter 5) showed fewer heart-disease deaths among the brothers remaining in Ireland, although they ate more cholesterol and fats. One of the reasons suggested for their better heart health was their greater physical activity. Other studies show similar results.

Dr. J. N. Morris of the London School of Hygiene has shown that bus drivers have two to four times higher incidence and greater severity of coronary heart disease than bus conductors, who walk and climb through the English double-decker buses (*Lancet,* 1953). The drivers and conductors surveyed had essentially the same diets, but the drivers averaged more than 15 pounds heavier.

Dr. H. A. Kahn made a similar study of mail clerks and mail carriers. The clerks had twice the incidence of coronaries as the carriers (*American Journal of Public Health,* 1963).

In general, if you work at a desk, you have twice the probability of a fatal heart attack as more active workers, according to a study of 192,000 men by Dr. Henry Taylor of the University of Minnesota (*American Journal of Public Health,* 1962).

Studies of high fat eaters who are very active people (such as lumberjacks in Finland, the Samburo and Rendille peoples of Kenya, and the Maasai of Tanzania) all showed that a physically active way of life reduces heart disease.

How Exercise Benefits Your Heart

The balancing of calories eaten with calories burned by activity produces arteries free of plaque, regardless of fat content of the diet. Additionally, vigorous activity produces larger artery diameters, to keep the blood flowing.

NASA studies show that an exercise program can result in a lower resting heart rate, lower blood pressure, increased stamina, better feeling of health, reduced weight, and reduced stress and tension. Furthermore, a study at the Cardiopulmonary Research Institute in Seattle found the mortality rate in heart patients not continuing a supervised exercise program was double that of patients continuing to exercise.

More recently, Dr. J. N. Morris has shown that vigorous exercise helps prevent heart attacks in executives. He studied 16,882 middle-aged male executives for two years. During the two-year study, 232 of the men suffered a first heart attack. Dr. Morris found that only 11 percent of those suffering their first heart attack engaged in regular vigorous exercise (89 percent of the victims did not exercise regularly). Of the remaining men not having an attack, 26 percent were found to engage in vigorous activity.

Dr. Morris concluded, "Vigorous exercise promotes cardiovascular health. Lighter exercise showed no such advantage. Habitual vigorous exercise during leisure time reduces the incidence of heart disease in middle age among male sedentary workers."

If blood cholesterol levels are important to you, consider the finding of Dr. Alfredo Lopez (Professor of Medicine at Louisiana State University), who observed that 10 weeks of vigorous exercise markedly lowers cholesterol levels.

The evidence presented in the studies quoted here is persuasive, but not absolutely conclusive. The June 1971 report from the National Heart, Lung, and Blood Institute Task Force on Arteriosclerosis advises, "The idea that regular physical exercise decreases the danger of death or disability from coronary atherosclerotic disease is based on a number of assumptions, some proven and some of questionable validity. . . . But there is no convincing data to indicate that exercise will, in fact, decrease either the rate of development of atherosclerosis, or prevent its complications."

Perhaps there isn't absolute proof, but there are lots of studies that show that, if proper precautions are taken, such as having a check-up with your physician first, progressing from oncy oxorcises to harder ones gradually, following tested programs and never overdoing it, exercise produces beneficial results that can be measured.

Dr. Ralph Paffenbarger and his colleages at the California State Health Department and the University of California at Berkeley have completed a 22-year study of 3,600 longshoremen in San Francisco with encouraging results. They found that a regular pattern of hard physical work nearly halved the risk of a fatal heart attack for the entire group of working men. The less active younger longshoremen ran a three times higher risk of suffering a fatal heart attack than those who worked hardest (*American Journal of Epidemiology,* March, 1977).

Exercise physiologist Jan Wallace (of San Diego State University) conditioned 16 men for 10 years, and all 16 (ages 42 to 66) remained free of heart disease.

Dr. Stewart Gorney (of the Longevity Research Center of Santa Barbara, California) found that many heart patients can improve within 30 days of supervised exercises to a point where heart-disease drugs are no longer needed. In some of his patients, angina was reduced 100 percent. In 75 percent of his patients, high blood pressure was normalized without drugs.

Dr. Gorney told a 1975 meeting of the American Academy of Physical Medicine and Rehabilitation that a controlled diet and exercise routine can "produce changes within a few weeks which increase blood flow and raise the oxygen content of the blood. The improved circulation quickly betters the patient's condition and permits the body to start the healing process that is the key to permanent recovery."

Physicians are actively debating whether the lifestyle of

a marathon runner can prevent heart attacks. One physician, Dr. Thomas Bassler, says he has never seen a report of a marathon runner dying of heart disease. Another physician, Dr. Lionel Opie, reported two cases of marathon runners having died suddenly (but there was, in these cases, no autopsy to establish heart disease). Although physicians debate the merits of exercise, few feel that our sedentary way of life is good for us. Personally, I doubt if I will ever run as much as marathon runners, but I do take large amounts of vitamins C and E, as many of them do.

Exercise Does Not Increase Appetite

If you are worried about eating more when you start an exercise program, rest easy. Controlled studies by Dr. Lawrence B. Oscat (Associate Professor of Physical Education at the University of Illinois) have proven that exercise does *not* increase the appetite. In fact, Dr. Brian J. J. Sharkey at the University of Michigan says that heavy exercise just before a meal can dull the appetite and cause caloric intake to fall below expenditure.

The One Exercise That's Good for Everyone

Just as there is biochemical individuality, the needs and ability of different individuals for exercise varies from person to person. Just as one person's meat is another person's poison, a form of exercise *just fine* for one person *may kill* another. There is only one exercise that I will strongly recommend for everyone. It's a daily deep-breathing exercise.

Regardless of the initial debilitating disease—heart disease, kidney failure, or whatever—most elderly persons actually perish from pneumonia. With age, lungs have a lower vital capacity than those of younger people, and as a result, lungs cannot handle the removal of debris and phlegm. This causes fluid accumulation, and when increased demand is placed upon the lungs, death results. A simple exercise done once a day will help maintain the required vital capacity.

The deep-breathing exercise can be performed sitting or standing, but standing is preferable. First, expel as much of the residual air in the lungs as possible by exhaling, then use your arms to further contract your lungs by extending your arms straight out and crossing one over the other as you bring them together. Continue the arm-crossing until the left arm is as far to your right side as possible and your right arm is as far to your left side as possible. Now expel the air with a whoosh as you lower both arms to your waist, while squeezing them "crossed" even more. This crumples your chest and lungs to expel a considerable amount of stale air. The extra squishing is good for body builders, but not required for older people who should stop prior to strain or discomfort.

Now relax your arms and straighten up while taking a good breath. Inhale as much as possible, while lifting your arms overhead and rising onto your toes. You should make another "whooshing" sound as a large quantity of air rushes in. Continue the upward stretch as far as possible. Then relax and breathe normally. This invigorating exercise can be repeated one to ten times if desired, but doing it once each day is sufficient to maintain vital capacity.

Exercise—Not Excuses

Don't just sit there listening to your arteries harden. The hardest part of the Total Protection Plan is thinking up excuses for not exercising. The exercise program for your heart takes little time, and actually becomes fun. Besides, your life depends on it!

Exercise and sex are both important to the heart patient. It is safe for heart-disease patients to exercise and resume sexual activities. The following chapter describes beneficial exercises for both the healthy and the recovering heart.

28

An Exercise Program
for Your Heart

Healthful exercise requires a *gradual* program in which activity is slowly increased. Young people in competitive sports may exercise to near strain, but that would kill or injure an older, out-of-shape person. One may, however, start an exercise program at any age. The best way to know what kind of exercise you can do is to have a physical examination during which a physician monitors your electrocardiogram while gradually increasing your exercise activity. Never decide to start jogging to get in shape without consulting your physician and having a thorough physical examination.

The next step is to listen to your body. Push it a little and see how it responds. Try to exercise at a level that increases your pulse by 10 to 20 beats a minute over your resting pulse. Try to sustain that increased pulse rate for 20 to 30 minutes. (You can take your pulse at either side of your neck on the muscle near the windpipe at one of the carotid arteries.) Stop before you are tired and see how long it takes to recover. Stop sooner if something seems wrong. Your pulse should fall at least 5 counts one minute after exercising. Repeat this level of activity three times a week for a month, and you will find that you have to exercise harder to get your pulse to speed up the 10 to 20 beats per minute.

The second month, you can try to exercise at an activity level that increases your pulse 20 to 30 beats a minute over a resting pulse. Your pulse should now fall at least 10 counts one minute after exercising. You can add more strenuous exercise each month as long as your pulse continues to fall at least 10 counts one minute after exercising and returns to normal in 10 minutes.

Progress in subsequent months by increasing your exercising pulse rate an additional 10 beats each month, until you reach the ideal exercising pulse rate given in Table 28.1. Remember, once a week won't do it. That may feel good, but it won't do your heart any good. Exercise three times a week, with a day's rest between days of exercise.

Table 28.1

Ideal Exercising Pulse Rates

Age	Ideal Exercise Pulse	Maximum Safe Rate
25	140–170	200
30	136–165	194
35	132–160	188
40	128–155	182
45	124–150	176
50	119–145	171
55	115–140	165
60	111–135	159
65	107–130	153
70	103–125	148
75	100–122	143
80	97–118	139
85	95–115	135
90	92–111	131
95	89–108	127
100	87–105	124

A reasonable goal for the 50-year-old would be a pulse of 120 for at least ten minutes, three times a week. Do not exceed a pulse of 220 minus your age at any age (and subtract another 30 beats if you have a heart condition).

The ideal exercising pulse rate is between 70 and 85 percent of the maximum safe heart rate. Incidentally, this corresponds to between 60 and 80 percent of the maximal aerobic power (maximum cardiopulmonary efficiency), which is a function of the consumed oxygen.

Don't forget that 5 to 10 minutes of gradual warmup must precede the exercise period, and 5 to 10 minutes of gradual cooldown, which includes walking about, stretching exercises, and a few calisthenics, must follow the exercise.

Begin with Moderate Activities

No matter how long it's been since you've exercised or even if you're recovering from a heart attack, there is a place to start from which you can progress to fitness. As an extreme example, you can begin by getting in and out of a chair repeatedly at a quick pace. You can stretch your muscles by standing up and swaying to music or dancing slowly. Next, you can try climbing stairs—just a few, and slowly at first. You may work up to bowling, playing table tennis, getting out of the house more, and walking briskly.

Even if it's been 5 or 6 decades since you were running around like a kid, and you lead a sedate life, you can still exercise to strengthen your body and improve agility. There are regular exercise programs given at many senior-citizen centers.

Choose Intermediate Activities That You Enjoy

When you are in half-decent shape, you can slowly take on more active exercise. What's best is to find an exercise that you like. I prefer basketball. You can play in your driveway or at a playground. You can shoot baskets by yourself, with friends, or play a game. You don't have to keep score and try to win to have a good time. You can play at whatever pace you wish. You will find yourself jumping, running, stretching, bending, and having fun. *Always do warmup exercises first.* Studies have shown that cold starts damage the heart.

Many people consider jogging, but it can be harmful. Jogging has in many cases brought on a heart attack or a frozen windpipe, which can occur when freezing air is inhaled through the mouth in deep breathing and can be fatal.

On the other hand, jogging has helped people reduce and keep in shape. If you are out of shape, jogging builds the heart and lungs, burns up calories, and builds leg, arm, stomach, and chest muscles, while massaging internal organs. It can be a beautiful experience if you jog where you can smell fresh air and flowers, rather than car exhaust fumes. **But jogging in a big city and inhaling large quantities of polluted air can be very harmful.** Jogging may or may not be good for you. Walking briskly, biking, playing tennis or golf, swimming, jumping rope, or running in place may be better.

Start a Daily Exercise Program

If your daily activity level is high, you need not exercise regularly except for enjoyment. But if you are sedentary, like most of us, an exercise program is a must.

The exercises you choose should include one to improve cardiovascular efficiency; that is, it should cause you to breathe hard. Other exercises should stretch your muscles and improve flexibility; still others should strengthen your limbs and trunk. Be sure to include leg exercises, as the contracting leg muscles squeeze the veins, thus helping return blood to the heart. Your exercise period should burn 300 calories daily. Consult Tables 28.2 and 28.3 to learn the calories consumed by common activities.

Whether Charles Atlas or someone else first recommended a daily dozen, the principle is still sound today. The following exercises are only suggestions. You are encouraged to substitute, add, or subtract to suit your objectives and conditions. If you have favorites of your own, make them part of your program. Do the following exer-

Table 28.2

Calories Consumed During Various Activities

Job Activity	Calories Used Per Hour	Recreation	Calories Used Per Hour
Answering		Badminton	400
telephone	50	Baseball	350
Bathing	100	Basketball	550
Bed-making	300	Boating, rowing	
Benchwork,		slow	400
sitting	75	Boating	800
Benchwork,		Boating, motor	150
standing	125	Bowling	250
Bookkeeping	50	Boxing	700
Brushing hair	100	Calisthenics	500
Brushing teeth	100	Card playing	25
Chopping a tree	480	Croquet	250
Dictating	50	Cycling, slowly	300
Dishwashing	75	Cycling,	
Dressing,		strenuously	600
undressing	50	Dancing, slow	
Driving truck	100	step	350
Driving tractor	150	Dancing, fast step	600
Dusting furniture	150	Driving a car	170
Filing (office)	200	Field hockey	500
Gardening	250	Fishing	150
Hammering		Football	600
(carpentry)	250	Golfing	250
Hanging up wash	270	Handball	550
Ironing	100	Hiking	400
Knitting	50	Horseback riding	250
Landering	200	Hunting	400
Mopping floors	200	Jogging	600
Mowing the lawn	460	Karate	600
Preparing food	100	Motorcycling	150
Reading	25	Painting	150
Sawing	500	Piano playing	75
Scrubbing floors	200	Running,	
Sewing	50	fast-pace	900
Shoveling	500	Shuffleboard	250

Sitting	70	Singing	50
Standing	80	Skating, leisurely	400
Stoking a furnace	675	Skating, rapidly	600
Sweeping floors	150	Skiing	450
Taking dictation	50	Soccer	650
Telephoning	80	Softball	350
Typing	50	Squash	550
Walking upstairs and down	800	Swimming, leisurely	400
Washing your face	150	Swimming, rapidly	800
Writing	50	Tennis, singles	450
		Tennis, doubles	350
		Volleyball	200
		Walking, leisurely	200
		Walking, fast	300
		Watching television	25

Data Compiled by the National Frozen Food Association

Table 28.3

Exercise—Calorie Equivalents

	Minutes			
Calories	Walking	Bicycling	Jogging	Swimming
100	19	15	10	12
200	38	30	20	24
300*	57	45	30	36

*Suggested daily exercise activity

cises only after you have passed the beginning stage. Generally, choose one or more exercises in each group. Switch to another exercise in that group periodically to prevent boredom.

Even during weeks when you are pressed for time, you should do at least one exercise every day (in addition to the breathing exercise mentioned in the previous chapter). And at least twice a week, do six different exercises in the same day.

Some Suggested Exercises

1. Back Stretch

   A. Bend and stretch—Stand erect, feet shoulder-width apart. Bend trunk forward and down, allowing knees to flex. Gently stretch and extend fingers to toes or floor. Return to starting position. Don't stretch too much on the first attempt. Gradually increase stretch with each repetition.
   B. Sitting Stretch—Sit on floor with legs spread far apart with hands on knees. Bend forward at waist, reaching fingers as far forward down each leg as you can with reasonable comfort. Return to start and repeat several times.
   C. Toe Touch—Stand with feet together. Bend trunk forward and down, allowing a slight knee flex. With a light bouncing motion, reach lower and lower until fingers touch toes (or as close as you can get). Return to start and repeat several times. Alternate with feet still together by stretching to the side of one foot and then to the side of the other.

2. Trunk Twist

   A. Body Twist—Stand with feet shoulder-width apart and arms extended outward from the sides, parallel to the floor. Twist upper body as far as possible with reasonable comfort to one side then the other, trying to twist a little bit farther each time. Turn neck at the same time. Repeat, but don't strain.
   B. Body Bend—Stand with feet shoulder-width apart and hands behind neck with fingers interlaced. Raise the left knee above waist height while twisting the trunk to the left and bend so that the right elbow touches the left knee. Return to starting position and repeat with right knee and left elbow. Keep fingers interlaced behind neck. Repeat several times on each side.

3. Stomach Strengthener

A. Upper Body Curl—Lie on back with hands tucked under small of back, palms down. Tighten stomach muscles, lift head, and pull shoulders and elbows up off floor. Hold for four seconds. Return to starting position and repeat.

B. Sit-Ups—There are many variations. Lie on back, legs together, arms extended beyond head. Bring arms forward over head while rolling up to sitting position. Touch toes with fingers. Roll back to starting position. Repeat. Alternate with bent knees or legs on incline. Also alternate with hands in back of neck and touching elbows to straight, bent, or alternate knees. You may hook your feet beneath a dresser or chair, if that helps you pull yourself up.

C. Alternate Leg Raises—Lie on Back. Lift straightened right leg off floor to a 45-degree position and hold for a second or two. Return to start and do it again. Repeat with other leg. Or alternately lift one leg and then the other in a swimming-kick motion.

4. Circulation—Strengthen Heart and Lungs

A. Run in place or skip rope.

B. Jumping Jacks (Straddle-Hop)—Stand at attention. Swing straightened arms upward from the sides until hands touch above the head, while simultaneously moving feet wide apart sideways in a single jumping motion. Spring back to starting position. Repeat several times.

C. Military Exercise (Squat Thrusts)—Stand erect, feet spread less than shoulder width, hands on hips. Do a full knee bend on toes with buttocks in air. Reach forward until hands touch floor. Shift body weight to hands while thrusting legs out straight behind. Spring back to knee-bend position, then return to standing position. Repeat.

5. Arm, Shoulder, and Chest Strengtheners

A. Arm Circles—Stand erect with arms extended sideward and parallel with floor. Rotate arms so that hands make small circles. Rotate one way for a while and then in the other direction. Try it with palms up and then with palms down.

B. Push-Ups—Lie on floor, face down, legs together, hands on floor under shoulders with fingers pointed straight ahead.

Push body off floor by extending arms so that body weight is on hands and toes (knees for beginners). Keep back straight and in line with straightened legs. Do not raise buttocks or let stomach sag. Lower the body until chest touches floor. Repeat several times.

C. Combination Exercise—Combine push-ups with the military exercise (4C). When legs are thrust back after the knee bend, you are in a perfect position to do a push-up and then resume the military exercise.

6. Leg and Buttock Strengtheners

A. Knee Bends—Stand with hands on hips. Bend knees (only halfway at first) while extending arms forward with palms down. Keep buttocks off floor. Allow heels to lift off floor and weight to roll to toes. Straighten up to starting position.

B. Squat—Similar to the exercise above, but keep feet flat on floor. Keep hands on hips throughout exercise.

C. Flutter Kick—Lie face down with hands placed under thighs. Arch the back by bringing chest and head up. Raise the legs up and kick as in swimming. Kick from hips with knees slightly bent.

There are countless more exercises. Some are figure exercises, some are endurance exercises, and some are strengthening exercises. If you can do all of those listed here, you are ready for advanced exercises, active sports, and even weightlifting. Seek out professional advice from your "Y" or health clubs. Excellent books abound on exercise. For exercises for men and weight training for men, women, and teenagers, I recommend *The Barbell Way to Physical Fitness* by Bruce Randall "Mr. Universe" (Doubleday, 1970). For women (both for health and figure exercises), I recommend the *21 Day Shape-Up Program* by Marjorie Craig (Random House, 1968). This book is especially good for women following pregnancy. Other fine books include *How to Keep Slender and Fit After Thirty* by Bonnie Prudden (Bernard Geis, 1969; Pocket Books, 1970), Olga Leiy's *Keep Moving* (Dial, 1973), and *Total Fitness in 30 Minutes a Week* by Dr. Laurence Morehouse and Leonard Gross (Simon and Schuster 1975; Pocket Books, 1976).

The Safe Way to Exercise after a Coronary

Many men fear that they can never be as active again or have active sex again after their heart attacks. The truth is that most men can be active in both. If exercise does nothing else, it gives heart patients a great psychological boost, returns them to happy productive lives, and dissipates the depression that follows heart attacks.

Heart attacks occur while at rest as often as while active. As indicated by the study by Dr. Arthur M. Master of New York City, 23 percent of heart attacks occur during sleep, 29 percent while at work, 24 percent during mild activity, 13 percent during walking at an ordinary pace, 9 percent during moderate activity. This percentage roughly equals the percent of time an individual spends each day on these activities.

Progress in exercising after a heart attack must be slow, gradual, and constant. Formerly, six to eight weeks of bed rest was prescribed after a heart attack. Now the patient is typically sitting up within three days, walking around his room in five to seven days, completely ambulatory after three weeks, and ready to exercise in two to three months.

Several studies have concluded that men recovering from heart attacks do not need to be less active in sex. There is no need to make changes in sexual position, time, or frequency. Of course, all published studies have been with wives or partners of at least six months, and some investigators caution about the added excitement or stress of a new partner. Even the stress of a new position is more harmful than activity, once you are reconditioned—so do what is most comfortable to you.

Although sex *can* be a vigorous life-prolonging exercise, a clinical study of coronary patients found that the average pulse rate during sex was less than that of walking or climbing two flights of stairs (H. Hellerstein and E. Friedman, *Archives of Internal Medicine,* 1970). The mean maximal heart beat during sexual intercourse is 117.4, which is less than the mean maximal heart rate during walking, climbing stairs, or various occupational activities. The psychological harm of not resuming sexual activity can be great (A. W.

Green, *New England Journal of Medicine,* 1975).

It is important for the partner to know there is no need to fear sex. As Dr. Harry Brody (of the Obstetrical-Gynecological Department of the University of Calgary) put it at a 1976 meeting of the Canadian Medical Association, "Wives of cardiac patients fear that sexual activity will precipitate another heart attack and have the additional nightmarish fantasy that the partner will die in the saddle."

Dr. Brody cautions against overeating or heavy drinking before sex, but advises that any patient able to briskly walk around the block is ready for sex. "The key point is that the cardiac patient can quickly learn to monitor his own functioning. If symptoms develop such as angina during a given activity, one should [in the future continue the activity, doing] everything and anything up to the point of producing these symptoms. The patient soon learns his own warning signals, what kinds of activities he can and cannot do, and how to stop short of producing pain. This is true for various kinds of exercise or resumed forms of sexual activity."

Some men actually say that they were thankful for their heart attack—not just because it taught them to appreciate life, which it did—but because they were forced to get in better shape. Now they are slimmer, stronger, more virile, and raring to go in activities that they had abandoned years before their heart attack. Now they are more admired, feel better than they have for 10 or 15 years, and have a better outlook on life. Other men have become semi-invalid after heart attack because of their fears—of having another attack. Generally after a heart attack, you can determine your destiny. Check with your doctor and when he approves, start exercising immediately.

29

Relaxation—Not Frustration

Stress contributes to heart disease in several ways, the most important being through the constant production of catecholamines (chemical hormones) that produce free radicals which can, in turn, cause artery cells to mutate and form plaques. Thus anyone living under constant stress is producing a constant excess of catecholamines that will lead to heart disease.

The word "stress" means different things to different people. We all seem to know it when we've got it, but just what we feel at such times varies from person to person. In order to cope with, or overcome, stress it is helpful to know what it is. The leading researcher on stress, Dr. Hans Selye (Professor and Director of the Institute of Experimental Medicine and Surgery at the University of Montreal, Canada), has defined stress as the nonspecific response of the body to any demand upon it. Certain biochemical "stress"-response reactions occur in the body regardless of the nature of the stimulus—pleasant or unpleasant. The "nonspecific" response Dr. Selye refers to is a demand for activity in the body to adapt to the stimulus.

Dr. Selye explains, "Stress is not simply nervous tension; stress reactions do occur in lower animals, which have no nervous system, and even in plants. Stress is not the nonspecific result of damage. We have seen that it is immaterial whether an agent is pleasant or unpleasant; its stressor effect depends merely on the intensity of the demand made upon the adaptive work of the body."

Although the concept of "stress" may seem confusing and technical, it boils down to the fact that persistent problems, which are or seem to be beyond our control, cause harmful chemical reactions to occur, if we allow our body to fight against the stimuli.

We can do two things to overcome stress. First, we can supply the body with an abundance of the specific nutrients required to handle stress. A subsequent section will specify those nutrients, and the Supernutrition Program in the final chapter will tell you how much and how often to take them. Second, we can learn how to relax rather than fight those problems that are beyond our control or influence anyway. If we don't do both, we may find ourselves developing heart disease.

Coronaries Are Linked to Behavior Patterns

Drs. Meyer Friedman and Ray H. Rosenman, cardiologists at San Francisco's Harold Brunn Institute of Mount Zion Hospital and Medical Center, studied behavior patterns and heart-disease incidence for more than 15 years, then published a book for the general public, *Type A Behavior and Your Heart* (Knopf, 1974), that explained the relationship.

Type A behavior occurs in a person with a high drive toward poorly defined goals, a persistence of work toward recognition and advancement, an eagerness to compete, and a heightened mental and physical alertness. Drs. Friedman and Rosenman define this behavior as "a special, well-defined pattern marked by a compelling sense of time urgency—hurry sickness—aggressiveness and competitiveness, usually combined with a marked amount of free-floating hostility." Friedman and Rosenman noted an unlucky 13 characteristics that they say point unerringly to Type A personalities, which make up about 50 percent of all Americans. Traits range from explosive accentuation of various key words in ordinary conversation and impatience with the speed at which things proceed, to a vague guilt feeling when they are relaxing—willingly or unwillingly. Such people are caught up in an aggressive and constant struggle to achieve more and more in less and less time. Type A personalities engage in polyphasic thought or performance (thinking about or doing two or three things at the same time) and, in consequence, they face heart disease anytime from the age of 20 on.

The Type B personality is not exactly the opposite. Type B individuals usually possess all the drive, intelligence, and ambition of Type A's, but they respond to challenges and time limits differently. A Type A person becomes irritated at having to solve a problem or overcome a challenge, while a Type B experiences increased security and confidence. The reason for this is that Type B personalities know their capabilities and limitations. Heart disease, according to Friedman and Rosenman, seldom strikes Type B's before 70, regardless of fatty foods eaten, cigarettes smoked, or lack of exercise.

In fact, Drs. Friedman and Rosenman found that 90 percent of their heart patients under 60 had Type A personalities. In 1960, they studied the personalities of more than 3,000 male volunteers aged 39 to 59. In a follow up 8½ years later, they found that the Type A's had had at least twice as many heart attacks as Type B's. They also discovered that a heart attack in a Type A person was twice as likely to be fatal as a heart attack in a Type B.

A confirming study came from Dr. C. David Jenkins of the Boston University School of Medicine. He studied the personalities of 2,750 men free of heart disease and followed them for four years to see which of them had heart attacks. The men who were rated high as Type A personalities turned out to have twice as many heart attacks (*New England Journal of Medicine,* 1976).

Dr. H. Pelser of Amsterdam studied 21 cases in which men had heart attacks before reaching 50 years of age. He found that all 21 had similar features in their personalities. They were vigorous, fearless, enterprising tough guys, respected by their fellow citizens and admired by any woman looking for an ideal partner. They worked harder than the average man, struggled for success, and felt guilty when they were inactive. In their effort to crush all competition, they were never able to play for sheer enjoyment. They would never openly admit defeat or frustration. They felt a need to dominate life and they substituted power for love. Obviously, these are not traits confined to men.

As early as 1959, Dr. Henry I. Russek identified emotional strain as a more serious heart-disease risk factor than diet, smoking, heredity, obesity, or lack of exercise. In examining 100 male heart patients under 40 years of age, he found 91 had experienced prolonged emotional strain associated with their work. He examined another 100 men under 40 not having heart disease, and found only 20 to have experienced similar stress. Among the heart-disease patients, 46 worked 60 or more hours per week, and an additional 25 were holding two jobs at the time of the attack. In the remaining 20, there was unusual fear, insecurity, discontent, frustration, restlessness, or a feeling of inadequacy in relation to employment.

An ongoing study of 1,000 medical students at Johns Hopkins over the past 30 years has found that most of the coronary victims, whether they had high cholesterol or not, were depressed, anxious, nervous, and angry under stress.

For those of you still concerned about blood levels of cholesterol, consider the following finding by Drs. Friedman and Rosenman. They checked the blood cholesterol levels of volunteer accountants from January to June. When the April 15 tax deadline approached, and their sense of time urgency rose sharply, so did the level of their blood cholesterol.

There are degrees of intensity in Type A behavior, and many people probably are a mixture of Type A and Type B. As women compete with men in business, they tend to become Type A's. The first step in alleviating Type A behavior is getting rid of the "hurry sickness" and learning to enjoy life as it is.

Learn how to recognize the situations that cause you stress, and practice physically relaxing your muscles before entering or during the stress situation. Relaxing methods include meditation, making your mind blank or thinking of pleasant scenes, going limp for a second, deep breathing, or relaxing muscles progressively, one at a time, starting with feet, legs, etc.

Culture and Coronaries

American men have one of the highest heart-disease death rates, while Japanese men have one of the lowest (the Japanese rate is approximately one-sixth that of the U.S. rate). Most researchers have long been convinced that the difference was due to diet, but a new study by Dr. M. Marmot and colleagues at the University of California at Berkeley seems to show that the real difference is cultural. The ten-year study found that among Japanese-Americans living in the San Francisco Bay Area, those who have become Westernized have 2 ½ times the rate of heart disease of those who continue to live a traditional Japanese lifestyle. Those who have become most removed from their culture have five times the rate found in the most traditional groups. In fact, they reach a rate as high as native Americans. The major difference seems to be in lifestyle and stress levels, as diet did not differ greatly among those Japanese-Americans in the Bay Area.

The traditional Japanese culture has built-in buffers to stress: individuals observe strict customs and rituals, and live in closely knit groups, in which there is greater emphasis on the group than on the individual.

Stress and High Blood Pressure

Stress doesn't cause high blood pressure in everyone—only in genetically predisposed individuals. (An estimated 5 to 15 percent of Americans are so predisposed.) Your inherited *tendency* for high blood pressure won't develop into high blood pressure until triggered by stress. Thus, even if you have hereditary essential hypertension, you can control it by minimizing triggering events or learning to defuse most of their explosive nature.

Most of the evidence suggesting that high blood pressure results from a combination of genetic susceptibility and triggering stress comes from animal research. Experiments by scientists such as Drs. Richard Friedman and Lewis K. Dahl of Brookhaven National Laboratory have shown that stress cannot induce high blood pressure in genetically immune mice, whereas it will in genetically susceptible ones.

Stress and Sudden Death

Severe stress can cause sudden death (rather than merely the formation of plaque in arteries or the development of high blood pressure). Often severe stress is better defined as "shock." We have all heard of people dying of broken hearts when the will to live leaves them. We have all known or read of cases in which, after the death of a person's mate of long standing, the survivor passed away within a month. Very likely, it was stress that killed the survivor.

In studies with dogs, researchers have found that irregular heart rhythms that can cause sudden death can be produced by mental stress (after the dogs' normal heart rhythms have been disturbed electrically). This implies, according to Dr. Bernard Lown of the Harvard School of Public Health, that, in those people with heart-rhythm abnormalities, mental stress can trigger sudden death. Dr. Lown has documented cases in which men have had their hearts go into ventricular fibrillation (rapid, erratic heartbeat) due to emotional stress although they have had absolutely no signs (hidden or apparent) of heart disease (*New England Journal of Medicine*, 1974).

How to Handle Stress

The best way to reduce the risk imposed by stress is by adding pleasure to your life. Learn to relax and enjoy. Although there are no studies that have conclusively shown that changing a Type A person to a Type B will actually reduce the risk of heart disease, it is certainly a prudent thing to do.

Learn to live a life of leisure by working at what you want to do. Enjoy the challenges and successes. Use the failures to learn, not to "burn." Manage stress and prevent distress.

Do useful things in your own way at your own speed. Don't try to eliminate all stress: some stress prevents boredom. Actors will put on boring shows if they don't feel butterflies before the opening curtain. Maintain your own level of stress at just the right tension level between boredom and distress. Make stress work for you and not against you.

Traditional methods of dealing with stress include the following steps: First, pay attention to your body and learn exactly what it is that makes you overtense. Are you angry? Do you grit your teeth, have cold hands? Are your forehead and neck muscles tense? Do your eyelids flutter? How about upset stomachs? What are your tension signs?

Once you recognize tension, the National Association for Mental Health suggests the following measures. Try a few of them.

1) Talk it out—don't bottle it up.
2) Work off your anger. Cool it for a day or two while expending physical energy in a do-it-yourself project around the house, playing tennis, or taking long walks.
3) Do something for others.
4) Escape for a while and come back prepared and composed.
5) Take one thing at a time in sensible priority.
6) Give in occasionally—even if you are right. This may lead to workable compromises.
7) Don't try to be Superman or Wonder Woman—be human.
8) Give the other person a break.
9) Go easy with your criticism.
10) Schedule recreation into your day's activities.
11) Make yourself available to other people. Volunteer and take the first step toward other people and new ventures.

Meditation and Biofeedback

Transcendental Meditation produces an extremely deep physical relaxation and reduction in anxiety. Dr. Richard Stone of the U.S. Veterans Hospital at La Jolla, California, tested 19 patients with high blood pressure and found that blood pressure was significantly lowered in more than half of the patients after several months of 15 to 20 minutes of meditation, twice daily (*New England Journal of Medicine,* 1976).

A Harvard Medical School study by Dr. Herbert Benson of 36 patients with high blood pressure found that meditation significantly lowered high blood pressure.

Meditation (or TM or Relaxation Response) essentially involves repeating a word (generally called a mantra) over and over until all thoughts, except occasional random thoughts, are out of your mind for a few minutes. Any one-syllable word, number, or nonsense syllable will work. The "universal sound," *Om,* is often used—so are the words *green, blue,* and *one.* Give it a try. Meditation is free and has no harmful side effects.

Nutritional Aids for Overcoming Stress

In situations of stress, the adrenal cortex is the most overworked gland. A person under stress must ensure that optimal levels of the water-soluble vitamins—the B-complex and vitamin C—are available in the bloodstream at all times. This may require taking "stress formulations" or other B-complex-with-vitamin-C preparations several times during the day (or taking sustained-release pills).

Sugar actually creates stress in the body, because it upsets the delicate balance between blood sugar and insulin. Cut down on sugar and you will cut down on stress. Smoking also creates stress, and if you smoke, you will need more of vitamins A, B complex, C, and E.

Pangamate (Vitamin B_{15}, discussed in Chapter 12) also helps the body deal with stress and normalizes blood pressure.

Well, just how bad is your frustration level, and can you lower it? Table 32.1, the Stress Index, in the final chapter, will help you measure your frustration level. Using the Stress Index regularly will help you chart your progress in dealing with the stresses of everyday living. Measure your frustration today. It's probably higher than you think, but with a little conscious effort and training you can lower stress and your risk of heart disease while raising your peace of mind and sense of pleasure.

30

Chelation Therapy—A Safe but Controversial Method for Freeing Your Arteries of Deposits

As long as we supply the body with adequate amounts of vitamins B_6, C, E, and choline, as well as the mineral magnesium, our arteries will not clog. But if our arteries are already clogged to an extreme state, it may be too late to free them of deposits with vitamins and heart-food supplements.

It is at this point that many undergo the risky and expensive coronary bypass operation. The technique involves diverting the flow of blood from a clogged artery through a section of vein removed from another part of the body and grafted to the coronary artery above and below the clogged portion.

Each year some 65,000 Americans have the bypass operation. One report shows that up to 12 percent of these patients die during the operation and subsequent hospitalization, that more than 10 percent die within a year after the surgery, and that within two years of the operation another 18 percent have died. Of the survivors, some 25 percent develop complications such as pulmonary embolism, pericarditis, pleuritis, and hemorrhage, and another 25 percent experience reclogging of the arteries within a year, thus facing the prospect of another bypass operation (E. D. Mundth and W. G. Austen, *New England Journal of Medicine,* 1975). In summary, up to 40 percent of those who have the bypass operation have died within two years; and 50 percent of the survivors have developed further problems. Still others are unable to have the initial or a subsequent bypass operation because clogged portions of critical arteries, such as the carotid (which supplies blood to the brain) are too extensive to yield to bypass surgery.

Fortunately, there is a safe, nonsurgical technique that with seeming magic flushes away the calcified deposits. This little-known procedure is essentially painless, and it works more rapidly than any alternative method. Originally called "chelation therapy," it is now often referred to as either "biotic therapy," "medical endarterectomy," or "chelation endarterectomy."

I do not mean to discourage a person from the bypass operation when it has been recommended by a physician. Most people feel better afterwards than they have in years. I only hope to point out that chelation therapy can be more effective and safer.

Previously another physician, Dr. Henry Russek of New York Medical College in Manhattan, remarked: "More lives are lost each year through bypass surgery on the heart than [are] saved by it. . . ."

Calcium Deposits Can Be Removed without Surgery

Chelation therapy has been employed for 25 years, but in the U.S. only about one thousand physicians practice it. It is not as glamorous or as financially rewarding for the physician as surgery, since it is quite a simple procedure.

First, a safe and inert compound (EDTA—ethylene-diamine-tetra-acetic acid) dissolved in solution is slowly introduced into the bloodstream. As the compound flows through the arteries, the hardened deposits of calcified material are removed from the arteries as though a powerful magnet were pulling out the rivets that hold a steel bridge together, or as though millions of microscopic magnets were extracting the calcium.

The EDTA doesn't, however, directly remove the calcium

250 Supernutrition for Healthy Hearts

from the clogged arteries. Actually, the chemical compound attracts and removes unbound calcium from the bloodstream, forcing the body to scavenge calcium from unwanted places, such as arteries, to resupply the bloodstream with calcium for transport to all of the body's cells.

As a result of the removal of calcium deposits, the cholesterol and other fatty substances in the arteries are softened and freshly exposed to the blood which metabolizes the now uncovered fatty deposits, breaking large molecules into smaller ones, producing energy and waste material in the process. Thus, clogged arteries are essentially freed of deposits.

EDTA does not dissolve the blood calcium bound to protein. Calcium in plaque, however, is loosely bound (electrostatically) and thus is readily mobilized into the bloodstream. Calcium in bone and teeth is not as readily mobilized because it is more strongly bound to protein. EDTA is administered slowly so that the hormone parathormone will mobilize only plaque calcium. After the EDTA treatment, the body's calcium supply is replenished by tablet supplements to insure that skeletal calcium is not mobilized afterwards. The calcium newly supplied to the blood does not, of course, go immediately into plaque, which forms over a long period of time.

Chelation therapy simply stated involves a change in the physical state of metastatic calcium (calcium in abnormal places). In the process, the solid calcium in deposits is dissolved into a liquid state, and thus can replace the unbound blood calcium that combined with EDTA and was subsequently passed out through the kidneys.

The chelating compound, which is administered as a liquid, must be introduced to the body slowly to prevent low blood calcium from developing, since the EDTA binds electrically charged (ionic) calcium. Approximately 45 percent of the blood calcium is in the unbound ionic state, while the remainder is transported bound to protein. Rapid administration of EDTA might result in hypocalcemia (low blood calcium), since it requires time for the parathyroid gland to respond to release the hormone parathormone which gathers calcium from deposits to compensate for the unbound blood calcium that combined with the chelating compound and is subsequently unavailable to the body. Low blood calcium is easily prevented by administering dilute concentrations of EDTA intravenously at a very slow rate over several hours, while the patient rests comfortably in a chair or bed. Since the patient is fully awake, he may read or watch TV, for the procedure is no more uncomfortable than giving blood.

Incidentally, the removal of a small amount of arterial plaque can result in a large improvement in blood flow. A law of fluid dynamics—Poisson's Law—states that if you increase the diameter of a tube by x, you increase the flow by x^4. Thus when you increase the diameter of an artery by 2 percent by removing plaque, you increase its flow by 16 percent.

It is important to realize that calcium deposits cannot be removed by simply avoiding calcium in your diet. This will not only fail to produce the desired effect, but will cause the serious disease of calcium deficiency, for calcium is required by the nerves for transmissions of impulses, muscle action (especially heart contraction), and the health of bone and teeth.

Russians First Reported Success with EDTA

My interest in the chelating compound EDTA was first aroused by reports in Russian scientific literature which claimed that the compound increased the lifespan of experimental mice by slowing their aging process. Conceivably, EDTA could have produced this effect on the aging process by removing excesses of metals, such as copper, needlessly deposited in skeletal tissue that would otherwise increase the rate of potentially dangerous free-radical formation. Because my earlier research had concentrated on preventing the damage caused by free radicals in the aging process, I followed the Russian research for a while with interest, although not with enough interest to initiate EDTA experiments myself.

Then EDTA caught my eye again. At a 1975 meeting of

the American Academy of Medical Preventics, I passed a poster exhibit by the president of the academy, Dr. Harold W. Harper of Los Angeles, who had displayed several infrared photographs (thermographs) of people during various stages of EDTA therapy. Because I had been involved with infrared photography, infrared spectroscopy, and infrared diagnostics for twenty years (initially as a college student), my curiosity got the best of me. Besides, I figured if anybody were attempting deception or if the physician were making any mistake, I would be able to spot it. After all, physicians are not trained in infrared techniques, and Dr. Harper could have been making mistakes in interpretation.

As I looked at the poster display, I became highly impressed by the thoroughness of his infrared calibrations, the legitimacy of the thermographs.

Although Dr. Harper and many others have shown the therapy to be safe and effective, *both the AMA and FDA attempt to prohibit its practice.* The poor reasoning that prompts them to do so will be examined in a subsequent section.

Chelation Is One of the Life Processes

Chemists use the term "chelate" (pronounced *key*-late) to describe the chemical complex formed between a mineral having two positive charges and a large organic molecule structured so that it holds the mineral with just the right amount of holding power. The chelate complex has different chemical properties than either the mineral or the chelating agent.

Chelation is a natural process that must occur in the intestine in order for most minerals to be transported through the intestinal wall. For example, when the inorganic mineral dolomite is taken as a food supplement, chelates are formed in the intestine in which the calcium and magnesium from the dolomite combine with the amino acids already present in the intestine. Only a small percentage of the calcium and magnesium dissolved by the stomach acid is able to be chelated and thus pass through the intestinal wall; eventually the unabsorbed portion is excreted.

The large organic molecules of amino acids which occur in protein can, and naturally do, form chelates with minerals such as calcium, magnesium, iron, zinc, copper, manganese, lead, and cadmium. In fact, only the proteins of these minerals that are chelated are able to be absorbed into the bloodstream.

While most of the inorganic forms of minerals that occur in mineral tablets pass through the digestive tract without being absorbed into the bloodstream, chelated minerals which occur in sources such as meats, vegetables, and fruits and in chelated mineral tablets are much more readily absorbed.

Other life processes such as digestion and enzyme production also involve chelation. For example, minerals are incorporated into chelates so that they can be digested. And minerals are released from chelates so that the molecules of enzymes can be built.

Since the removal of material from within an artery is called "endarterectomy," chelation endarterectomy refers to the removal of minerals or metals from within the artery by means of chelation.

Chelation Therapy Is Now Safer Than As Originally Practiced

Perhaps Dr. Norman Clarke, a physician with a private practice in Detroit, was the first to experiment with chelation therapy in 1948. Since that time, the procedure has been modified extensively, but the chelating agent of choice remains EDTA. Since EDTA is inert, it does not enter into any reactions in the body (other than by attracting unbound ionic minerals), nor does EDTA, once in the body, break down into other compounds.

Fifty percent of the administered EDTA is excreted in the urine within the first hour, 90 percent within 4 hours, 98 percent within 6 hours. No organ except the skin retains

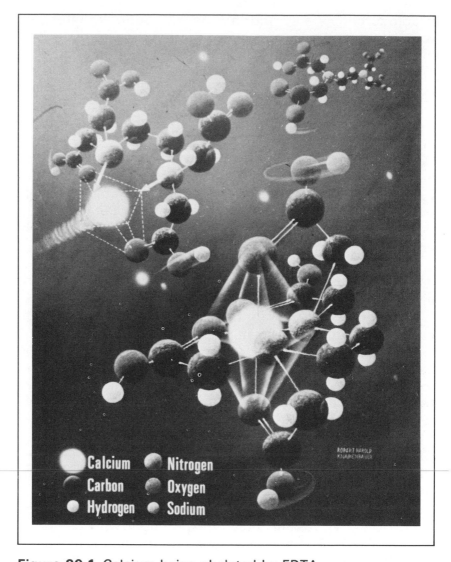

Figure 30.1 Calcium being chelated by EDTA.
Original drawing by R. Harper. Reprinted with permission of the copyright owner, Dr. Harold W. Harper.

more than 0.5 percent of the EDTA after 48 hours, an amount harmful to no one, yet beneficial to patients having scleroderma, a progressive disease of the connective tissue.

Presently, U.S. physicians are administering about one-tenth of the EDTA dosage used for chelation therapy in 1948. In 1953, a death was attributed (perhaps falsely) to too-rapid administration of 26 grams of EDTA within 24 hours. Since then, treatments have been given in series, normally 2 to 7 days apart. The physician will decide the best treatment schedule for each patient.

As a precaution, mineral concentrations in the patient's urine are monitored closely before, during, and after treatment, and the patient today is given mineral supplements following each treatment in order to compensate for amounts carried away from the blood by EDTA.

It is reassuring to know that calcium is the mineral primarily removed by EDTA because of the pH level of the blood. Other minerals less effeciently removed are first the toxic minerals—lead, cadmium, mercury, and nickel. Thereafter, the EDTA binds zinc, magnesium, copper, manganese, cobalt, iron, and chromium.

A number of sessions are required in the course of chelation therapy, but once the treatment is completed, the patient's disease state is usually altered for one to six years. If new deposits form, the treatment can be repeated.

A single treatment with chelation therapy costs between $40 and $60, and since the average patient requires from 20 to 30 treatments, the total cost is generally from $1,000 to $2,000. The cost of an arterial bypass operation, by contrast, varies from $15,000 to $60,000. Those who argue that insurance covers the bypass operation should realize that insurance contributes only 80 percent, leaving the patient to pay the remaining $3,000 to $12,000. Unfortunately, no insurance covers the cost of chelation therapy. Remember, it's not accepted by the AMA.

The benefits of the risky bypass operation last no longer than, if as long as, those of chelation therapy. In the past 30 years there have been a number of highly touted new heart operations, none of which has met expectations. The bypass operation first performed in the Cleveland, Ohio, Clinic in the mid-1960s offers improved blood supply. The published medical literature shows that 23 percent more of the patients who survive the by-pass operation will be alive

5 years after treatment than those not given surgery. After five years, however, the survival rates are essentially the same. But it is important to realize that those given surgery are the healthier patients, many claiming to feel better than they have in years (E. D. Mundth and W.G. Austen, *New England Journal of Medicine,* 1975).

The relief from angina (heart pain) these patients' experience may be entirely due, however, to the severing of the pain-receptor nerves to the heart as a result of the surgical incision (Ross, *American Journal of Cardiology,* 1975).

A point often overlooked is that when tests indicate a slight deterioration in artery health—that is, when reclogging has started—it is a simple matter to pursue a minor course of treatment such as chelation therapy before the damage is extensive.

Still, chelation therapy, according to Dr. Harold Harper, has significantly helped 90 percent of those refused bypass operations because of being poor risks.

In commenting on the surgery, Dr. Eliot Corday (of the University of California at Los Angeles) observed in 1975, "We still don't know the first fact—whether bypasses increase survival. We simply don't know how long the graft will last." "It's just a fad based on emotion, experimental interest, and prestige," claims Dr. George Burch of Tulane University Medical School. And Dr. Reginald Hudson (of Grady Memorial Hospital in Atlanta) remarked, "My private opinion is that they will go out of fashion in five years." (All quotes are from syndicated copy by David Zinman in *Newsday.*)

Surgery is always a drastic measure, and requires that you wait until your condition has become serious. Yet most of those who survive the bypass operation must face similar surgery every two to four years.

"More lives are lost each year through bypass surgery on the heart than have been saved by it," according to Dr. Henry Russek (Professor of Cardiology at New York Medical College in Manhattan). "Fifty-five to sixty percent of these die during the operation or within a year of it. Or they suffer heart attacks which result in their becoming permanently disabled." Dr. Russek estimated that during the course of the some 65,000 bypass operations performed each year, up to 30 percent of the patients experience some kind of heart attack on the operating table. "Those who recover from the initial heart attack are still left with myocardial infarction, which is the very condition that bypass surgery was designed to prevent." (*Time,* March 4, 1974)

Drs. L. Griffith, S. Achuff, and their associates at the Johns Hopkins University Medical School determined that a significant number of occlusions occur in coronary arteries after bypass surgery, thus impeding blood flow. This result was confirmed by six other groups of researchers (Gina Kolata, *Science,* 1976). Specifically the Johns Hopkins group found that 40 percent of the arteries had new occlusions just six months after the surgery.

Also at Johns Hopkins, Drs. B. Bulkley and G. Hutchins, who studied 97 bypass operations, were dismayed to find problems within a day or two. They report: "The causes of fibrin platelet thrombi in the native arterial tree are many, and may also apply to transplanted veins. Almost any factor which damages the vascular endothelium may result in deposition of thrombi on its surface. Surgical manipulation, stretching due to arterial pressure, and changing blood flow patterns may disrupt vein endothelium and precipitate microthrumbus formation. Whatever the original insult, however, our findings indicate that intimal mural fibrin do form in the majority of vein grafts within 24 hours of implantation and continue to form for months. That at least some of these thrombi undergo the usual course of organization into a plaque is difficult to dispute . . . and the development of the early atherosclerosis in these transplanted veins is highly probable."

Although most people with angina experience immediate relief after surgery, this relief may be temporary. Dr. E. Alderman of the Stanford University School of Medicine found that 40 percent of 350 patients had recurrence or worsening of pain within 2 to 5 years after surgery.

Dr. M. Platt of the University of Texas Health Center found evidence of newly damaged heart muscle in 31 percent of the patients.

Dr. A. Rosati of the Duke University Medical Center studied 490 people who underwent the bypass surgery and 611 equally diseased patients. He found that surgery did not help the mortality rates of these groups.

The Veterans Administration cooperative study has found no differences in mortality rates of the medical and surgical groups.

In 1972, Dr. D. Brewer, also of the Duke Center, had reported that one in five patients undergoing the surgery had myocardial infarction on the operating table (*Journal of the American Medical Association,* 1972).

In addition to the success of chelation therapy in preventing heart attacks, secondary benefits from EDTA therapy arise as a result of the removal of calcium deposits, because the freshened-up areas can now absorb magnesium and zinc normally, thus improving nutrition in tissues formerly "starved." Neither a balanced diet nor vitamin supplements can produce thoroughly beneficial effects unless the absorbed nutrients are able to reach all regions of the body.

Because chelation therapy, or even large amounts of vitamins C and E, remove deposits and improve circulation, such damage as senility and the blindness associated with severe diabetes, once thought irreversible, can sometimes be repaired.

The full beneficial effect of chelation therapy is not felt until 60 to 90 days after treatment. Although my explanation of why this occurs sounds rather technical, it is at least brief. The reason is that the EDTA removes metal ions from the lysosomal membranes of each cell in which those membranes have become "poisoned" or clogged. When the membranes are clogged, the lysosomes (scavenging enzymes) are hindered from passing through into the cell interior (cytoplasm). Consequently, the lysosomes are restrained from properly flushing the cells and, as a result, the cells no longer are efficient. After chelation therapy, a gradual process occurs during which lysosomes regain the ability to fully flush cells, thus increasing cellular efficiency and restoring health to normal. Improvement in the patient's health usually continues for 2 to 4 months after the treatment as the body heals itself because the blood channels have opened. At that point, proper vitamin supplements (such as those suggested in the Total Protection Plan and Dr. Rinse's Breakfast) can keep new deposits from forming.

The Benefits of EDTA Therapy Can Be Measured

The extent of the improvement is immediately obvious to the patient, and can be readily confirmed by several diagnostic tests. The use of infrared thermographs is an especially clear way to monitor the progress of chelation therapy. As thermography alone cannot tell the whole story, it is used in addition to more conventional clinical tests, including x-rays and blood tests.

Basically, in thermography, an infrared (heat-ray) photograph of the patient is taken under controlled room temperature. Warmer areas of the body will appear on the photograph as brighter or whiter colors, while cooler areas will appear darker. The significance of the differences revealed is that the areas not receiving the normal amount of blood are cooler and can be readily spotted as dark areas on the infrared photograph.

If, for example, one of the carotid arteries (which go from the aorta to the head) is partially blocked, then one side of the face will be slightly cooler than the other, and show darker on the thermograph. By contrast, the presence of cancer will produce a bright area because cancers are generally "hot spots" of chemical reactions that release heat. Thermography is consequently becoming an important tool in routine examinations for breast cancer. Even very small areas of warmer or cooler temperature, such as a small region above the eye, can be easily spotted.

Dr. Harper's "poster lecture" contained several sets of thermographs, each showing the improvement in circulation that resulted from chelation therapy. Indeed, the results were dramatic, and there was evidence that the improvement did continue after the final administration of EDTA.

EDTA Therapy Attacked by Medical Establishment

Medical literature throughout the world contains many accounts of amazing cures brought about by chelation therapy. Much of the progress in the United States has been brought about by physicians who have practiced the therapy such as Drs. H. Spencer, J. F. Holland, C. P. Lamar, N. E. Clarke, A. Soffer, M. Seven, H. M. Perry, R. S. Guber, S. A. Muller, L. Meltzer, T. N. Pullman, A. Weinberg, R. Evers, and P. Williamson, and more recently, G. Gordon, B. Holstead, R. Vance, and H. Harper.

Yet the technique is avoided by a U.S. medical establishment that prefers surgery, although in difficult cases surgery cannot compare with the success of chelation therapy. Furthermore, surgery cannot reach all the places chelation therapy can. Bypass operations cannot, in most cases, be performed in the kidney, neck, or brain.

For just one example, consider the following 1975 report by writer Tom Valentine in the *National Tattler:* "Gregor Milne, 54, of Catalina Island, suffered a massive heart attack in 1965. He flew to the famed Houston clinic of Dr. Michael DeBakey, internationally known specialist. After five days of testing, Dr. DeBakey told Milne: 'We know what you have, but don't know how you got it, and don't know how to get rid of it. There is a general buildup of deposits around your heart and there is no place to cut. Therefore, I can't help you.' Milne said he was put out to pasture [by other physicians] on a low-cholesterol diet. 'I barely existed, always in pain for three years.'

"After nine days of chelation therapy with a chelating physician, Milne noted dramatic improvement. He claims to be a whole new guy."

An editorial in a following issue of the *National Tattler* revealed that the newspaper had received a tremendous response to the article, perhaps greater than for any other article they had carried. The article had discussed the fact that the therapy cures arthritis and prevents heart attacks. Those claims caused the AMA to prosecute the doctor as a "quack," in spite of the more than 18,000 documented case histories of successful EDTA therapy from his own practice and the practice of another physician that the doctor had available for the AMA's examination.

California health authorities were convinced that the AMA's claims of quackery were justified, and placed charges against the doctor that were brought to court in 1974. According to the newspaper's article, the case was thrown out of court when the doctor and more than a thousand patients prepared to prove the effectiveness of the treatments.

Harassment of physicians who practice chelation therapy has not been restricted to the physician involved in the California court case.

At the 1975 spring meeting of the American Academy of Medical Preventics, where I saw the "poster lecture" by Dr. Harper, I was invited to attend several podium lectures on chelation therapy. The first speaker was, however, unable to appear because legal harassment by state authorities prompted by the medical establishment had interfered with his preparations for the lecture. Fortunately another speaker, available to teach the procedure in his place, was well received as he traced both the progress of chelation therapy and the AMA harassment of those practicing it.

A sample of the anti–chelation-therapy opinion from Dr. Alfred Soffer was revealed by Tom O'Neill in the *National Bulletin* in 1976. Dr. Soffer (who heads the American College of Chest Physicians in Chicago) pointed out that the AMA's Committee on Quackery has declared against EDTA. "About 15 years ago," Dr. Soffer explained, "this treatment was investigated by scientists including myself, but after a series of studies no result came of it. Eventually all research stopped and most of us forgot about it. Then suddenly, we discovered that a strange fad had started up—the cult of the 'new wonder drug.'

"One clinic has described the treatment as 'often lifesaving and sometimes miraculous.' Any miraculous cure probably resulted from a wrong diagnosis in the first place."

Personally, I believe Dr. Soffer has closed his mind to the progress that has occurred since his research 15 years ago.

The method of administration has changed, mineral supplementation is now given, new clinical tests have been added to monitor the chemical activity, and infrared photography is currently used to verify both the diagnosis and progress. Perhaps if Dr. Soffer visited a modern clinic using chelation therapy, he would again become enthusiastic about this dramatically effective technique. He was originally an advocate of chelation therapy when he wrote the chapter "Chelation Therapy for Cardiovascular Diseases" in a book he edited titled *Chelation Therapy* (Thomas, 1964).

Dr. Thomas Ballantine (Chairman of the AMA Committee on Quackery), who reviewed the reasoning for banning chelation therapy in that same *National Bulletin* article, stated: "This is not an established method of treatment." And in 1966, the AMA Council on Drugs said, "The drug [EDTA] is not useful in the disease [atherosclerosis] because none of the beneficial effects is lasting."

Here we have a veiled admission that in 1966 there were beneficial effects, although our attention is drawn to a concern over the duration of the benefits. Yet even the "new" arteries formed during bypass operations eventually become clogged (generally within two years after the operation).

No studies have yet been conducted comparing the benefits of chelation therapy with the benefits of nonintervention and surgery, although the National Heart, Lung, and Blood Institute is now starting such a study comparing the effectiveness of the bypass operation with nonintervention. With over 1 million Americans dying annually from heart disease, it's time that the AMA updated its 1966 opinion of chelation therapy.

Research Funds Should Be Granted

Research funds should be made available to further refine chelation therapy, for it seems to me that chelating agents that can be taken orally could be found. For example, the natural amino acid cysteine is an excellent chelating agent and readily passes through the intestine into the blood-stream. (EDTA, by contrast, is a synthetic organic compound.) I do not know if cysteine will bind calcium as well as it does lead, but the medical establishment needs to know. It's time the medical establishment began looking for improved chelating agents and stopped harassing practitioners.

Since the profit from this treatment is comparatively low and the harassment high, I had wondered what made a few physicians persist in the treatment when they could have opted for official sanction and the more profitable treatments. After hours of discussions with a number of them, I have concluded that once they realized how many people could be significantly helped, they believed the treatment should be made available to all those wanting it. I found that, almost without exception, the physicians employing chelation therapy have had the treatments themselves. In addition, many have treated members of their families.

The most often repeated criticism of chelation therapy by the political medical establishment has been that no scientific data are available, and that no double-blind study has been done to prove the efficacy of the therapy. Yet when I visited the offices of the American Academy of Medical Preventics, I found an astonishing number of published scientific papers with an abundance of information concerning chelation therapy. The copies of the published material, which contained numerous reports of positive results of chelation therapy in humans, filled two standard file drawers. These were only the articles published in English. Additional articles are published in many languages, including Russian and the languages of many of the Eastern-bloc European nations. During a trip to Russia in 1976, I found chelation therapy to be a conventional technique and, interestingly, the Russians give credit to the original observations of Dr. Norman Clarke and other American researchers.

As for double-blind studies, they involve the administration of a treatment to one group of patients and an inert placebo to another group. The problem in conducting double-blind studies of chelation therapy is that those in the untreated control group run the risk of dying. The critics should observe that until recently there had not been a double-blind study on bypass surgery, for the same good reason.

The only scientific article negative to chelation therapy was published by Dr. J.R. Kitchell of Philadelphia (*Lancet,* 1961). Interestingly, only three weeks prior to this publication, Dr. Kitchell (one of the original researchers in the use of chelation therapy, when large grants were available) had made an announcement along with Dr. L. Meltzer, in *Medical World News,* to the effect that chelation therapy was the greatest thing on the medical horizon.

Curiously the conclusions of Kitchell's subsequent negative article cannot be supported by the data within the article. In the beginning of the article it is stated that all of the patients were hopelessly ill, while later in the same article it is noted that 40 percent of these same patients remained free of symptoms more than four years after chelation therapy. The conclusion was that chelation is not lasting and is of questionable value. Perhaps those 40 percent freed of all signs of heart disease after having been declared "hopeless" would have a different view.

How to Locate a Doctor Who Practices Chelation Therapy

Widespread use of chelation therapy would be of immense health benefit to the 65,000 people who annually undergo the coronary bypass operation. And the availability of the therapy would considerably ease the financial burden that their heart disease creates.

The pharmaceutical-hospital-medical cartel which escalates the cost of care beyond the capability of the American people to pay would be the loser. But those who pay insurance premiums (which contribute 80 percent of the cost of bypass operations) would be the winners.

Chelation therapy can be administered by any family physician, internist, or cardiologist with very little expensive equipment. All tho physician needs is an intense desire to learn, a few weeks of special training, and an experienced office staff.

It is estimated that there are 900 to 1,200 physicians using chelation therapy in the United States. If you wish to locate the doctors in your area who treat atherosclerosis with chelation therapy, write to the American Academy of Medical Preventics, c/o Mrs. Lynne Stone, Executive Vice President, 9201 Sunset Blvd., Suite 912, Los Angeles, California 90069, and enclose a self-addressed, stamped envelope for their reply.

I have talked with patients who have had all three coronary arteries mostly blocked with plaque and were encouraged to undergo triple bypass operations, but who opted for chelation therapy instead. They were free of symptoms within 6 to 8 weeks after the conclusion of the therapy and were still free of symptoms when I spoke with them over a year later.

I have read case histories of patients so weakened that they arrived at a clinic in a wheelchair or on an ambulance stretcher, only to leave as normal after several weeks of chelation therapy.

Chelation therapy is definitely suggested for the person with life-threatening atherosclerosis. Those with a more moderate condition may "rinse away" their plaques with a breakfast comprised of special supplements, as detailed in the next chapter.

31

Dr. Rinse's Breakfast for Freeing Your Arteries of Deposits

Most of us have some cholesterol deposits in our arteries. If the degree of atherosclerosis is immediately life-threatening, I suggest chelation therapy. If the degree of atherosclerosis is mild to moderate, I suggest optimum nutrition, which I call Supernutrition (explained in details in the final chapter). However, if your arteries are moderately to severely clogged with plaque, then it is advisable to speed up the Supernutrition process with a proven supplement often called the Rinse Breakfast.

The Rinse Breakfast was developed by Dr. Jacobus Rinse of East Dorset, Vermont, as a convenient way to take several of the special "heart foods" that I discussed in earlier chapters.

I first learned of the Rinse Breakfast in 1971 when Dr. Rinse and I began corresponding about nutrition and the aging process. Dr. Rinse told me that his breakfast brew seemed to produce a synergistic effect between the various vitamins and minerals. It was becoming widely known in Holland, because he had lectured there on the subject and the diet produced such remarkable results.

In late 1972, he reported that he was receiving many more confirmations of the value of the Rinse Breakfast, with some of the reports very striking and clinically controlled. Physicians remarked that they had never seen such improvements and complete disappearance of deposits. I suggested to Dr. Rinse that he publish the breakfast and his experience with it in *American Laboratory*, a scientific magazine read by 90,000 U.S. chemists, medical researchers, and biologists. His article appeared in the July 1973 issue, and parts of the article are reproduced here with the permission of *American Laboratory*.

In June 1974, Christine Jukes reported on the Rinse Breakfast in *Prevention*. So many readers thereafter commented on the benefits of the Rinse Breakfast that Dr. Rinse was asked to write more details and experiences in the November and December 1975 issues.

The success of the breakfast was so enthusiastically reported by readers that Jane Kinderlehrer and the *Prevention* Fitness House staff developed additional variations of the Rinse Breakfast to aid those who didn't like to eat cereal for breakfast every morning or didn't like the taste of the special "heart foods." They published additional recipes (see Appendix 7) for Dr. Rinse's pancakes, wheatless granola, Dr. Rinse's omelet, bran muffins, and two variations of a spread for bread in the April 1976 issue of *Prevention*. A reader also reported that the ingredients could be blended into vegetable or tomato juice.

Dr. Rinse had been struck with heart disease in 1951, even though he had been following all of the rules for reducing the risk of heart disease as promoted by the American Heart Association. At this writing, he is 77 years old and free of all signs of heart disease.

Here is Dr. Rinse's own account, condensed from *American Laboratory*.

An attack of angina pectoris in 1951 at the age of 51 initiated an inquiry by me into possible reasons for the occurrence of atherosclerosis. Starting with an hypothesis that deficiencies in my food could be causative factors, dietary changes were explored, resulting eventually in the complete alleviation of angina and related heart diseases. This paper describes the evolution of the successful dietary changes, explores details of the hypothesis, and cites some recent work supporting important aspects of the hypothesis.

Following the 1951 attack of angina pectoris with attendant violent heart aches, the attending heart specialist predicted that I might have another 10 years to live if all physical exercise was avoided. I was completely puzzled, because in my case none of the known causes was valid. I did not smoke, was not overweight, had no special tensions, had sufficient physical exercise, and had no family history of the disease.

Personal Experiences

These started in 1951 at the age of 51, with a gradually increasing pressure or light pain in the breast after increased exercise. In the beginning, the sensitivity disappeared immediately after the physical activity ended, but during a hike against wind and uphill, pain began when I did not stop, and I had a severe heart ache which made me nearly faint. Although the pain diminished when I stopped, the light pressure in the breast remained for several days, also during resting. A heart specialist diagnosed angina pectoris and prescribed anticoagulant (Dicumarol) and nitroglycerol tablets.

After the pressure in the breast had disappeared in a few days, I began to work again, but avoided heavy physical activities. Also I stopped using anticoagulant. However, walking up a staircase or a hill always reminded me that the angina was still there, because my pulse increased strongly to become normal only after one hour.

The suspicion that a food deficiency caused the trouble brought me to experiment with enzyme-rich food, such as raw herring, raw eggs, red meat, uncooked vegetables, yogurt, etc. It is difficult to conclude whether there was any effect. However, the use of garlic definitely increased the activity limit.

Food Supplements

In the meantime, I began to use one gram of ascorbic acid (vitamin C) per day, because earlier I had good experiences with it for curing and preventing colds and flu. Later a multivitamin pill was added. My breakfast consisted of a cereal with milk and yogurt, fortified with wheatgerm, yeast, and brown sugar (one tablespoon of each). When I read an article about two Canadian physicians (Drs. Shute, London, Ontario) who treated heart patients with tocopherol (vitamin E), I asked their advice and they prescribed 200 mg vitamin E after each meal. I used these additives for several years and, by avoiding strenuous exercise, I managed to live a more or less normal life with only occasional warnings that the angina pectoris was still present. I always worked until the pressure in the breast warned me to take a rest. Also, the pulse rate was used as a control. Early in 1957 and later in October of that year, I experienced attacks with heavy heart pains, which subsided after an hour or so. The angina pains remained after the second attack, especially walking up stairs. At the same time, spasms and an increase of 60 strokes in the pulse rate were observed frequently.

Because the possibility existed that allergy might cause the angina, I checked this with the pulse rate and found no effect. At that time I read about a series of experiments with rats and rabbits who got lecithin or safflower oil, with the result that the cholesterol content in the blood was lowered. I decided to add a tablespoon of each to my cereal breakfast, which contained the other additives also.

Results appeared in a few days because the spasms stopped and the increased pulse rate diminished slightly but definitely. The improvement continued until after three months all symptoms of angina pectoris, even after exercising, had disappeared. One year later, the capacity for heavy outdoor work and running had returned. This result seemed to be too good to be true, and in the beginning I would not believe it. But it appeared to be a fact, because I have had no recurrence of angina or other diseases since—now 16 years later.

More Experiences

Following the advice of a Dutch physician (Dr. W. L. Ladenius), I put my experiences in writing and gave copies to people who were interested. In December 1960 a colleague, Dr. W., who had survived a cerebral thrombosis and a heart infarct at the age of 53, decided to take the food supplements. One half year later he was again working full time and he has had no relapse since. He is convinced that the breakfast has helped to cure him. At the same time a 69-year-old executive of Dutch industries (S.) had a blood clot in one of his legs, used anticoagulants, and followed strict diet without eggs or butter. Learning about my experience he cured himself rapidly and even has started a new industry. Because he considered safflower oil the most important supplement, he made a fat containing a mixture of highly unsaturated oils, palm kernel fat, and nitrogen as a substitute for butter. It is now widely used in Holland.

After a second chemist (Dr. W.) also found his condition improved with the breakfast, we wrote a short note for the Dutch paper *Chemisch Weekblad,* titled "Is Atherosclerosis Reversible?" Shortly afterwards, *Chemical Week* (in U.S.A.) published two of my letters to the editor about the same subject. The results of this publicity began to spread a year later in several letters, mostly from people we had not met. One letter written by a man of 72 years (J.) who suffered from a series of heart attacks and angina pectoris explained how he cured himself in three months' time and was able to take long walks again, which had been impossible during six years. Another letter was from a Dutch mechanical engineer (R.) who, at the age of 48, had such severe angina pectoris that he had to stop working and found no relief by drugs prescribed by several heart specialists. He did not believe that our breakfast could help him, but after insistence of a friend he tried it and was back to work in two months' time. He can run again, and works at times in deep-freeze storage rooms without any bad effects. A 72-year-old consulting chemist (W.) from Texas had suffered from heart attacks, read the letter in *Chemical Week,* and improved rapidly. He stopped using the prescribed medicines and is again at work. A lady of 70 years (Mrs. P.) in Manchester, Vermont, had survived blockings in the neck artery and partial paralysis. In December 1967 she started with the food supplements, which tasted exceedingly good to her. Her health improved rapidly and she has had no recurrences. Clinical tests showed that all cholesterol deposits had disappeared. Numerous similar cases could be cited.

Besides those individual reports, I received an invitation to meet a Dutch internist (Dr. K.) and I saw him in May 1963. He told me that he prescribed the breakfast to numerous older patients with spectacular results. Many of them had resumed their activities, even after having been invalids for a long time. Six years later, Dr. K. was still enthusiastic about the supplements.

From other correspondents I learned that a beginning cataract disappeared after the patient used the diet additives; this happened to two elderly ladies. A colleague (K.) wrote me that he regulated his wife's blood pressure with what he called "Rinse's Morning Feed." A chemical engineer (B.), who had worked in the sugar factories on Java, immediately accepted our advice with the comment that he had cleaned blocked pipes in his factory with phosphoric acid, and that therefore lecithin, being a phosphate, might be effective for his heart condition. He indeed cured himself and ten years later was still in good health. In 1969, a man from Chicago (P.) wrote that he had cured himself of arthritis, and two friends of bursitis, by using the food supplements. At present several thousands of people in Holland and U.S.A. and some in England and Belgium use the above supplements, although most physicians ignore the method. Only some of them advise patients not to use them.

Modifications

It is not necessary to use all of the ingredients at the same time in a breakfast. Each person can make variations suited to his taste and need. The most important components are lecithin and polyunsaturated oil, but the other products may be necessary. In any case, they cannot do any harm. Some people cannot eat yeast without stomach disturbance. In that case, more vitamin B complex is recommended. Instead of combining the additives with milk or yogurt, one may add them to fruit juice or to soup. One colleague (A.) adds wheatflour, and bakes cakes that are quite tasteful. Quantities may be varied, and less than a tablespoon can be used when all symptoms of atherosclerosis have disappeared. It is convenient to mix all dry components and make a supply for one month. Polyunsaturated oil can be used by way of a soft margarine, or it can be used on salads. Besides the previously mentioned ingredients, the use of finely ground bone meal is recommended as a source for calcium, magnesium, phosphate, and trace metals.

Since the breakfast was developed, several papers have appeared confirming various aspects of the working hypothesis. Some important corroboration comes from studies of cholesterol.

Cholesterol Content

Although statistically the chance for atherosclerosis is higher if the cholesterol content of blood is high, many persons are healthy with a high cholesterol content. This has been discussed by van Buchem in his publications. Therefore it is doubtful whether the efforts to lower cholesterol content by all means are justified. Such efforts include avoidance of food containing cholesterol such as eggs and butter, or using drugs that affect the production of cholesterol in the liver. It has been demonstrated that the liver produces more cholesterol if food contains less. Reducing its production by the liver by means of drugs can be dangerous and has caused serious side effects, such as cataracts and the loss of hair. It seems that one cannot change cholesterol production in the body without penalty. On the other hand, if lecithin is added to the diet, the unwanted deposits of cholesterol derivatives do not form, because the lecithin-cholesterol compound is soluble. Both materials occur in eggs, and therefore an atherosclerotic patient should not deprive himself of eating eggs. We have seen that polyunsaturated oil should be present. Any excess of cholesterol in the bloodstream is removed from the body through the intestines. . . .

The diet should contain lecithin in sufficient amounts. Lecithin occurs in nuts, seeds, eggs, and soybeans, and is produced in commercial quantities from soybean oil. The linoleate content depends upon the climate and the geographical source. The technical product contains other phospholipids. Lecithin and other lipids are hydrolyzed by metabolism into smaller molecules, which pass through the intestinal wall and reconvert into lecithin in the liver. Because the great majority of fatty acids in human food are of the saturated type, chances are that the lecithin produced in the liver will contain these fatty acids in larger quantities. Therefore, the addition of some polyunsaturated oil (linoleates) simultaneously with lecithin is desirable to obtain low melting derivatives. The daily requirements of lecithin and polyunsaturated fatty acids are of the same order as those for cholesterol, being a few grams per day. The molecular weight of lecithin being about twice that of cholesterol, one needs 4–6 g of lecithin and an equal amount of linoleate per day. If, however, a condition of more or less advanced atherosclerosis exists, the amounts of lecithin and oil should be increased. Morrison prescribed the previously mentioned amount of lecithin for his patients three times per day. However, some patients could not tolerate this much, and therefore lesser amounts may be indicated. Linoleate is also an intermediate for the production of the prostaglandin hormones.

The consumption of polyunsaturated oils by themselves (without lecithin) would not be effective, as one can conclude from the preceding consideration. Only in the presence of sufficient lecithin can the polyunsaturated fatty acid help in dissolving cholesterol. In countries with high fish consumption, such as Norway, the addition of polyunsaturated oils alone did not have any effect. It is lecithin that they need. It is understandable that van Buchem after an extensive investigation reaches the following conclusion: "The advice to recommend the consumption of polyunsaturated oils by the whole population with the exclusion of saturated fats is insufficiently founded."

Is atherosclerosis reversible?

This question, which we discussed in 1961 in *Chemisch Weekblad* and in *Chemical Week,* now can be answered affirmatively. At least less severely stricken and younger patients appear to have been cured completely without restriction of normal physical activity. This means that the cholesterol deposits in their blood vessels have been solubilized, and the narrowing has disappeared. The same has happened with older patients (65–80 years), and they felt relief and resumed activity. However, if their arteries have already lost flexibility or contain weak spots and calcium deposits (arteriosclerosis), then they should be cautious not to strain themselves so as to prevent internal hemorrhages. Several cases have been reported. After full recovery from atherosclerosis, physical activity is desirable to train heart, lungs, and other organs, and to help prevent recurrence of atherosclerosis.

The recommended and proven natural products to be used are soybean lecithin, wheat germ, brewer's yeast, and bone meal, available as powders or grains or flakes, which can be mixed and stored indefinitely, provided light is excluded. A practical ratio is 4:4:4:1, and daily requirement is only 15–25 g (two tablespoons) of the mixture. It may be consumed with milk or with fruit juice or with soup. A polyunsaturated oil (five grams) should be added, and finally these natural additives should be supplemented with synthetic (or natural) vitamins C and E and a multivitamin-mineral tablet. If sugar is desired, the dark brown quality or molasses syrup or honey should be used.

Although I have concentrated on finding a cure for atherosclerosis, I have learned that the food supplements also have been helpful in several other diseases, such as colds, flu, infections, arthritis, bursitis, and backache. It is probable that they also prevent these troubles, based on my experience. Several correspondents have written to me about such effects.

Food Supplement for Prevention and Cure of
Atherosclerosis

The following combination of natural and synthetic vitamins and minerals has proved to be beneficial for the cure and prevention of atherosclerotic complications, such as high blood pressure, angina pectoris, cataract, obstructions in the arteries of neck, legs, arms, and kidneys. Consequently, heart infarcts and cerebral thrombosis become avoidable.

A mixture is made of one tablespoon each of soybean lecithin, debittered yeast, and raw wheatgerm and one teaspoon of bone meal (ash). (It is recommended to prepare a larger quantity for storage.)

Mix in a bowl:

Two tablespoons of the above mixture, one tablespoon of dark brown sugar, one tablespoon of safflower oil or other linoleate oil, e.g., soybean oil. [I recommend *no more* than this.—R.P.]

Add milk to dissolve sugar and yeast.

Add yogurt to increase consistency.

Add cold cereal for calories as needed or mix with hot cereal such as oatmeal or porridge. Raisins and other fruits can be added as desired.

For severe cases of atherosclerosis, the quantity of lecithin should be doubled.

Indeed, Dr. Rinse's Breakfast does work to rinse away plaque from clogged arteries and promote a sense of well-being. It is not a diet—only a breakfast—that many people will find pleasant-tasting and convenient to use. There is little practical value in a food supplement that will not be used due to inconvenience, taste, or expense.

If you are one of the few people who do not enjoy a cereal for breakfast, use your imagination to create your own way of combining these important food supplements.

Dr. Rinse's Breakfast works because it puts Supernutrition to work. Other dietary regimens work well too. Since we are all different, one system of supplementation will not be preferred by all. General improvement has been achieved in some people with high-protein, low-carbohydrate diets (Dr. Robert Atkins, *Dr. Atkins' Diet Revolution,*

Bantam, 1972) and others with a high-carbohydrate, low-fat diet (Nathan Pritikin, *Live Longer Now,* Grosset & Dunlap, 1976).

Remember that any *balanced* diet will help the body heal itself and reverse the third stage of plaque formation. Just how do you know if your diet is balanced? Take the Supernutrition Quiz and follow the Supernutrition Plan explained in the next chapter

32
The Total Protection Plan

In preceding chapters, the various functions of specific vitamins and minerals in helping to prevent or cure heart disease have been described. The Total Protection Plan, however, includes more than supplements of these vitamins and minerals. It requires exercise, calorie balance, abstinence from (or severe reduction of) smoking, and control of stress and blood pressure.

It's easy to chart your progress toward your goal of a super-healthy heart. Calorie balance can be checked with a bathroom scale. Blood pressure can be monitored in free neighborhood clinics or at home. Exercising pulse rate can be measured by a clock with a second hand. Cigarettes can be counted. And stress level can be determined with the aid of Table 32.1. Checking your progress in optimizing vitamin and mineral supplements involves spending only two or three minutes at two-week intervals answering the first fifteen questions of the Supernutrition Quiz (p. 289).

Of course, you may use the guidelines for dosages of specific vitamins given in individual chapters, but, since those suggested amounts represent standard levels and each of us is biochemically individual, better results may be obtained by tailoring dosages to your needs.

Table 32.1

Stress Index
An index of your frustration level—Try to
progressively lower your index.

Activity	Decreased	Same	Increased
A			
1. Number of arguments			
2. Times doing 2 or 3 tasks simultaneously			
3. Rushed or skipped meals			
4. Restless nights			
5. Late for, or missed, appointments			
6. Instances of automobile speeding or catching up to the car in front of you			
7. Missed opportunities to tell your family and friends how much you appreciate them			
8. Missed opportunities to help someone else			
9. Glances at the clock			
10. Indigestion or stomach upset			
11. Times interrupting others			
12. Missed opportunities to totally relax or meditate			
13. Times gritting teeth or fidgeting			
14. Periods of hostility			
15. Number of criticisms of others			

Score 0 points for each "decrease" answer, 5
points for each "same" answer, and 15 points for
each "increase" answer.

Activity	Decreased	Same	Increased
B			
1. Non-work-related activities			
2. Time spent with family and friends			
3. Periods of meditation or short naps			
4. Long walks			
5. Time spent listening to others or reading			

Score 0 points for each "increase," 10 points for
each "same," and 20 points for each "decrease."

Table 32.2 provides a Progress Chart to help you monitor your progress toward total protection against heart disease. You should check your progress at one-week intervals for the first three months, then at intervals of two weeks for the next six months. Thereafter, check your progress at three-

Table 32.2

Total Protection Plan Progress Chart

Antioxidant Nutrients	(Increase Supernutrition Score or maintain good level)
	It isn't necessary to take the Supernutrition Quiz every week. Take it every other week and simply carry over your score for the following week on your progress chart below.
Blood Pressure	(Decrease or maintain good level)
	Those who have had heart disease or high blood pressure or are over 50 should check their blood pressure at least once a month after they have been on the program for 9 months.
	See Table 22.1 for indication of good levels.
Cigarettes	(Decrease or maintain low level)
Diet	(Decrease weight or maintain good level)
	And eat a well-balanced diet at all times.
Exercise	(Increase or maintain good level)
	Exercise level should challenge your pulse rate.
	See Table 28.1 for indication of good exercising pulse rates.
Frustration	(Decrease Stress Index score or maintain low level)

Table 32.2 (cont'd)

	Antioxidant Nutrients	Blood Pressure	Cigarettes	Diet	Exercise	Frustration
1						
2						
3						
4						
5						
6						
7						
8						
9						
10						
11						
12						

Your heart can now be 5 years younger than when you started the Plan

14						
16						
18						
20						
22						
24						
26						
28						
30						
32						
34						
36						

Your heart can now be 10 years younger than when you started the Plan

1 Year						
1¼ Years						
1½ Years						
1¾ Years						
2 Years						

The Progress Chart is a record of your success in following the Total Protection Plan. Give yourself a plus (+) or a minus (−) for each of the six steps—A, B, C . . . D, E, F—each week for the first three months. For the next six months, check your progress at intervals of two weeks. From this point on, continue to check your progress at intervals of three months. If you maintain good levels in each of the six factors, your heart will not only grow younger and stronger, but stay younger and stronger.

month intervals. The results of your progress checks, which you record on your Progress Chart, will give you guidance in the fine tuning of your own Total Protection Plan.

Your frustration level, which is recorded in column F of the Progress Chart, can be determined with the help of the Stress Index (Table 32.1). The Supernutrition Score, which is recorded in column A of the Progress Chart, is explained in the following pages.

The Supernutrition Score

To measure your progress in the Total Protection Plan, you will need a quantitative measurement of your present health so that you will know where you are at the start and if you are improving or maintaining good levels as the weeks pass. You will need a physical examination for certain health measurements and to detect any valid organic reasons as to why you should not take certain vitamins and minerals—e.g., serious kidney disease or metabolic defects. The quantitative measurement is called the Supernutrition Score and the means of determining your score is with the Supernutrition Quiz and Scorecard.

The quiz is merely three series of questions that you use to measure your body's performance. One series of questions of major importance determines 40 percent of your Supernutrition Score. These questions concern a combination of subjective and objective measurements. The second series of questions is mostly subjective but allows you to note the subtle improvements you might otherwise miss. The final series of questions can be answered only through an examination by your physician. The examination will provide an independent objective measurement to insure that you are making real progress and are not doing harm to yourself. It will remove all doubt.

You determine your Supernutrition Score by answering each question and putting a check in the appropriate box on one of the Supernutrition Scorecards (Figures 32.1–32.3). After filling in the proper boxes corresponding to your present condition, you convert the boxes into a numerical score by using the instructions immediately following each series of questions. You record your score on the Supernutrition Scoreboard (Figure 32.4), which becomes your permanent reference.

After two weeks on the Supernutrition program, you repeat the procedure, recording your second score in the "2 weeks" portion of the Scoreboard, and noting your improvement. You repeat the process at two-week intervals until you have reached your highest consistent Supernutrition score. This is the score you will try to maintain to keep yourself in the best of health.

A Word of Caution

Some people invariably become overinvolved or worry about their physiological measurements. Physicians often hesitate to tell patients what their blood-pressure or blood-chemistry values are because these patients worry themselves needlessly. Yet an informed person can keep the values in perspective and use the information constructively. Please be informed that because of biochemical individuality and other genetic differences, many people with blood-chemistry values above the range considered "normal" for the majority of people have perfect health. Therefore, deviations from "normal" do not always indicate a problem. The purpose of the Supernutrition Scoreboard is to monitor the *trend* of your blood chemistry and general health to see if you are improving with increased vitamin consumption or not.

You might also worry needlessly because your blood pressure or blood chemistry doesn't fall into the best category of the Supernutrition Scorecard. If you are not yet in superior health, you still may be in far better health than 80 percent of the people considered "healthy." The scorecard is designed to give, on a "weighted" basis, increasingly higher points for the better values, and few if any points for values just outside of average. Therefore, an "average" person will have a very low score, not far above a "sick" person's score. The *trend* of the Supernutrition Score is higher as a person reaches his or her best values, whatever they may be.

Figure 32.1 Instant Score—If you can spare only a minute right now to assess your present health, this is the score card to use. The highest total possible is 200 points (180 if you don't include the blood-pressure question). To find your percentage of relative health, which is independent of disease, blood-chemistry values, and long-term factors (such as resistance to colds), divide your *instant* Supernutrition Score by 2 (or multiply by 0.5). If you didn't include the blood-pressure question, divide by 1.8 (or multiply by 0.6). *Your* best health may be reached at a value somewhat less than 100 percent.

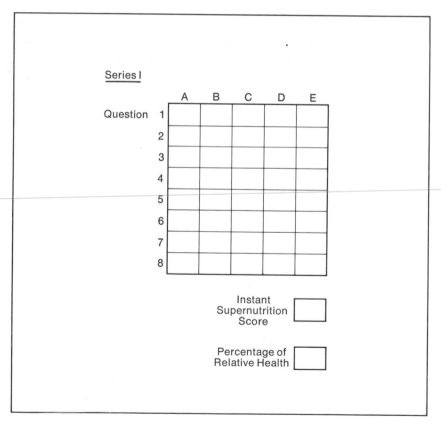

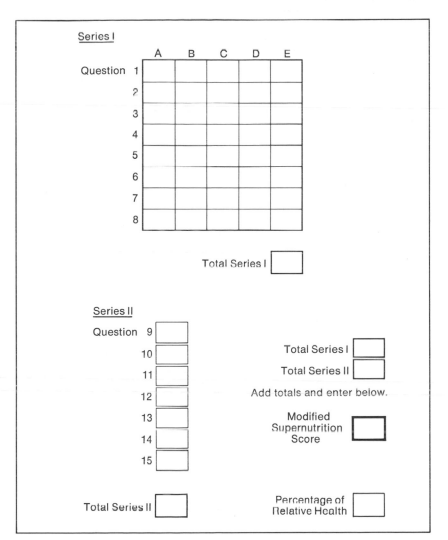

Figure 32.2 Modified Score—If you can spend two or three minutes for a fuller survey of your present health, but do not have the results of a recent physical exam, use this scorecard. To find your approximate short-term percentage of relative health, which is independent of disease, blood-chemistry values, and long-term factors (such as resistance to colds), divide your *modified* Supernutrition Score by 3.6 (or multiply by 0.28). If you did not include the blood-pressure question, divide your score by 3.4 (or multiply by 0.3). A Modified Supernutrition Score of 360 (without blood pressure, 335) represents the approximate best "variable" health for an average person. *Your* best health may be reached at a lower value.

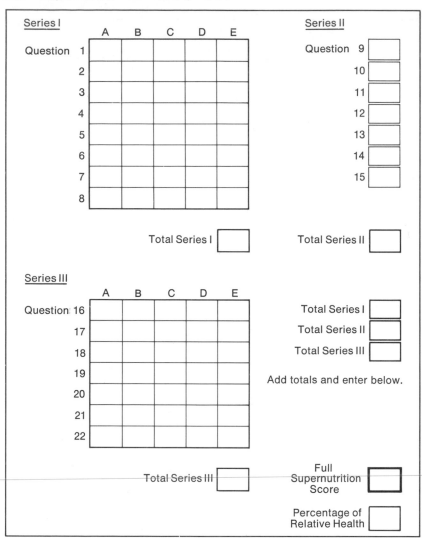

Figure 32.3 Full Score—If you have the results of a recent blood analysis and urinalysis, use this scorecard to find your Supernutrition Score. To find your short-term percentage of relative health, which is independent of disease and long-term factors (such as resistance to colds), divide your *full* Supernutrition Score by 5 (or multiply by 0.2). A perfect Supernutrition Score of 500 indicates 100 percent of the best "variable" health for the mythical "normal" person. *Your* best health may be reached at a somewhat lower value.

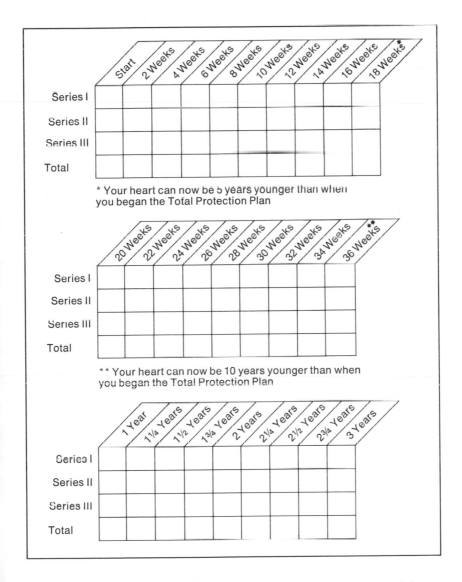

* Your heart can now be 5 years younger than when you began the Total Protection Plan

** Your heart can now be 10 years younger than when you began the Total Protection Plan

Figure 32.4 Record your Supernutrition Score at two-week intervals for the first nine months and at three-month intervals thereafter.

A third needless worry may be the tests themselves. Many people experience anxiety when they have their pulse or blood pressure taken, thus increasing heartbeat and blood

Instant Score (questions 1–8)	Modified Score (questions 1–15)	Full Score (questions 1–22)	Percentage of Relative Health	Interpretation
192–200	346–360	480–500	96–100	Superior Health. You probably practice Supernutrition.
182–191	328–345	455–479	91–95	Good Health. Your health can improve noticeably.
172–181	310–327	430–454	86–90	Average Health Plus. Most will benefit significantly from Supernutrition.
162–171	292–309	405–429	81–85	Average Health. You probably need Supernutrition badly.
152–161	274–291	380–404	76–80	Less than "average" health, but not necessarily "poor" health. You will notice a rapid improvement with Supernutrition.

Figure 32.5 Your Supernutrition score will monitor the progress of your health as you follow the Supernutrition program. Because of biochemical individuality (differences in genetics, activity, etc.) everyone in the best of health will not reach the highest scores. What is more important than your score is the protection the program gives you against heart disease and the improvement you notice in the way you feel. Take the Supernutrition quiz (beginning on page 289) at the intervals suggested by the program and enter the results on your Supernutrition scoreboard. To understand how well you are progressing, compare your score with the ones given here.

pressure. As you get used to taking these readings, your anxiety will disappear. Try resting for a few minutes before taking them, and immediately before taking them, take two (and only two) deep breaths. If your readings are high, don't worry, because you are now starting a program that will improve them.

Women should not attempt to find their Supernutrition points while pregnant.

The only three physical measurements you need to make for the Instant or Modified Supernutrition Score, which will indicate your present level of health, are weight, pulse rate, and blood pressure. If you don't know your present blood pressure, you can still determine your Instant or Modified Supernutrition Score. Of course, you should get your blood pressure checked just as soon as you can, unless your last (and recent) reading was within normal range. (See page 171.)

Monitoring Your Weight

I assume that you weigh yourself regularly. Compare your weight to the "ideal" weight listed in Table 32.3 to find your percentage variance from the ideal. The simple calculation is as follows:

Step 1: Subtract your "ideal" weight from your present weight. (If your present weight is the same or less than your "ideal" weight, enter a check in block A of question 8. Otherwise proceed to step 2.)

Step 2: Divide your ideal weight into the difference that you obtained in step 1. Multiply this answer by 100 to convert to percentage. Check the appropriate block in question 8.

Example:	Step 1:	present weight	168
		ideal weight	140
		difference	28

$$\begin{array}{r} 0.20 \\ \text{Step 2:} \quad \text{(a) } 140\overline{)28.00} \end{array}$$

(b) $0.20 \times 100\% = 20\%$

Table 32.3

Weights for Men and Women Aged 25 and Over (in pounds according to height and frame, in indoor clothing)

	Height feet	inches	Small Frame	Medium Frame	Large Frame
	(1-inch heels)				
MEN	5	2	112–120	118–129	126–141
	5	3	115–123	121–133	129–144
	5	4	118–126	124–136	132–148
	5	5	121–129	127–139	135–152
	5	6	124–133	130–143	138–156
	5	7	128–137	134–147	142–161
	5	8	132–141	138–152	147–166
	5	9	136–145	142–156	151–170
	5	10	140–150	146–160	155–174
	5	11	144–154	150–165	159–179
	6	0	148–158	154–170	164–184
	6	1	152–162	158–175	168–189
	6	2	156–167	162–180	173–194
	6	3	160–171	167–185	178–199
	6	4	164–175	172–190	182–204
	(2-inch heels)				
WOMEN	4	10	92–98	96–107	104–119
	4	11	94–101	98–110	106–122
	5	0	96–104	101–113	109–125
	5	1	99–107	104–116	112–128
	5	2	102–110	107–119	115–131
	5	3	105–113	110–122	118–134
	5	4	108–116	113–126	121–138
	5	5	111–119	116–130	125–142
	5	6	114–123	120–135	129–146
	5	7	118–127	124–139	133–150
	5	8	122–131	128–143	137–154
	5	9	126–135	132–147	141–158
	5	10	130–140	136–151	145–163
	5	11	134–144	140–155	149–168
	6	0	138–148	144–159	153–173

Source: Boehringer Ingelheim, Ltd., Elmsford, N.Y. 10523

Monitoring Your Pulse Rate

To determine your pulse rate, take a reading at your wrist or neck for a full minute. The full minute will give you the accuracy needed to differentiate between the closely grouped values in question 7. The full minute will also give you time to become at ease while taking the measurement. Be sure that you haven't been exercising or moving around much during the fifteen minutes preceding the measurement; it is not valid to compare your pulse rate after sleeping with that after walking upstairs. Your scorecard is meaningful only if conditions are constant, and reproducible each time.

The Supernutrition Quiz

If you can spare only a minute right now to assess your present health, answer only questions 1–8. Choose only one letter for each question; enter a checkmark in the appropriate box on the Instant Supernutrition scorecard (Figure 32.1). If you can spend two or three minutes for a fuller survey of your health, answer questions 1–15, using the Modified Supernutrition scorecard (Figure 32.2). If you have the results of a recent blood analysis and urinalysis, answer questions 1–22, recording your answers on the Full Supernutrition scorecard (Figure 32.3).

Series I. Major

1. Blood pressure (normals from 90/60 to 140/90). (If not known, leave question 1 blank.)
   Is your blood pressure:
   a) 120/80 or less
   b) between 121/80 and 125/85
   c) between 126/85 and 140/90
   d) between 141/90 and 165/95
   e) above 165/95

2. Energy level
   Do you normally feel:
   a) peppy, zesty
   b) alert
   c) average
   d) tired, sluggish
   e) exhausted

3. Mood
   Are you:
   a) thrilled with life
   b) happy
   c) average, OK
   d) blah
   e) depressed, moody

4. Stamina
   Is your endurance:
   a) excellent
   b) good
   c) average
   d) fair
   e) poor

5. Bowel regularity
   Are your bowels:
   a) very regular
   b) mostly regular
   c) almost regular
   d) poorly regular
   e) constipated

6. Headaches
   Do you have headaches:
   a) no more than once or twice a year and mild
   b) seldom
   c) occasionally
   d) often
   e) often and severe

7. Pulse rate (after 15 minutes of rest; normals 65 to 90, average 75)
   Is your pulse rate:
   a) below 65
   b) between 65 and 70
   c) between 71 and 75

    d) between 76 and 85
    e) above 85

8. Obesity
   Is your body weight:
   a) less or the same as "ideal" weight (according to Table
      32.3)
   b) less than 10% above "ideal"
   c) between 11 and 15% above "ideal"
   d) between 16 and 20% above "ideal"
   e) more than 20% above "ideal"

Total the number of checks under each letter. Multiply by the following factors: 25 points for each *a* answer, 15 points for each *b,* 10 points for each *c,* 5 points for each *d,* and zero for each *e.* Enter your total at the bottom of the Scorecard. Maximum score for Series I is 200.

Series II. Subjective

9. Chronic pain
   Answer yes or no:

sinus	yes	no
back	yes	no
neck	yes	no
eye	yes	no
shoulder	yes	no
elbow	yes	no
finger	yes	no
when urinating	yes	no
muscle cramps	yes	no

   Give yourself 1 point for each "no" answer (maximum 9 points). Enter total here＿＿.

10. Swelling
    Answer yes, reduced (since the last time you answered the question), or none:

face	yes	reduced	none
hands	yes	reduced	none
ankles	yes	reduced	none
joints	yes	reduced	none

    Give yourself 2 points for each "none" answer and 1 point for each "reduced" (maximum 8 points). Enter total here＿＿.

11. Skin, hair, and nails (Improved refers to the time since you last answered the question.)

	Column a	Column b	Column c
skin	smooth	improved	rough
veins showing in face	none	reduced	yes
veins showing in legs	none	reduced	yes
nails, color	normal (pinkish)	—	discolored or pale
hair, condition	glossy	—	dry and brittle
hair, amount	normal or regrowing	—	balding
hair, color	normal or returning	—	graying
eyes	bright and clear	—	dull or red (blood vessels)
circles under eyes	none	reduced	yes
bruise easily	no	—	yes

Give yourself 2 points for each answer in *Column a* and 1 point for each answer in *Column b* (maximum score 20). Enter your total here_____.

12. Oral

	Column a	Column b	Column c
gums	healthy	improved	diseased
tongue, color	normal	—	pale or red
tongue, surface	normal	—	rough or swollen
breath	odorless	—	halitosis
mouth sores	none	improved	yes

Give yourself 2 points for each answer in *Column a* and 1 point for each answer in *Column b* (maximum 10 points). Enter score here_____.

13. Circulation
Answer yes or no:

leg cramps, restless legs, intermittent lameness (especially at night or after walking)	yes	no
shortness of breath	yes	no

tightness in chest	yes	no
cold feet or hands	yes	no
hands or feet "go to sleep" easily or become numb	yes	no
muscle twitches	yes	no
extreme sensitivity to weather changes	yes	no

Give yourself 3 points for each "no" answer (maximum 21 points). Enter your score here_____.

14.1 *For females only*

Answer yes or no:

	Column a	Column b
irregular periods	yes	no
premenstrual tension or premenstrual depression	yes	no
painful menses or painful breasts	yes	no
menopausal hot flashes	yes	no

14.2 *For males only*

Answer yes or no:

prostate trouble	yes	no
frequent night urination (after bedtime)	yes	no
dribbling or difficult urination	yes	no
sexual staying power	not as desired	as desired

Give yourself 4 points for each answer in *Column b* (maximum 16 points). Enter your score here_____.

15. Miscellaneous

	Column a	Column b
dizziness or fainting spells	yes	no
buzzing or ringing in ears	yes	no
allergy	yes	no
cough (chronic)	yes	no
indigestion or heartburn	yes	no
weakness if meals delayed	yes	no
hard stools	yes	no
poor appetite	yes	no
nausea	yes	no
trouble sleeping	yes	no
stiff joints	yes	no
hemorrhoids	yes	no

diarrhea	yes	no
urine (does not refer to color but to transparency)	cloudy	clear
urination frequency	more than six times daily	six times daily or less
reflexes	slow	fast
vision	blurred	clear
sex, enjoyment	average or poor	good or excellent
sex, frequency	less than first 2 years of relationship	same or more than first 2 years of relationship

Give yourself 4 points for each answer in *Column b* (maximum 76 points). Enter score here_____.

Total score for Series II, questions 9–15 (maximum 160 points). Enter on your scorecard.

Series III. Medical
Some clinical laboratories may use different analytical procedures for these tests and thus provide different "normal ranges." When you ask for your test result, also ask for the normal range for that laboratory. If the normal range is different than indicated here, merely adjust the values here for each choice proportionally.

16. Blood pressure (normals from 90/60 to 140/90). (Enter again even if answered in question 1.)
    Is your blood pressure:
    a) 120/80 or less
    b) 121/80 to 125/85
    c) 126/85 to 140/90
    d) 141/90 to 165/95
    e) above 165/95

17. Cholesterol (normal values 149 $\pm$ 36)
    Is your blood-cholesterol level:
    a) 175 or lower
    b) 176 to 200

c) 201 to 235
d) 236 to 275
e) above 275

18. Triglycerides (normal values 10 to 200, or your age plus 110; values can go to 4,000)
Is your blood triglyceride level:
a) 100 or less
b) 101 to 150
c) 151 to 200
d) 201 to 300
e) above 300

19. Hematocrit (normals: men, 47 $\pm$ 7; women, 42 $\pm$ 5)
Is your hematocrit:
a) 40 to 43.9 (men)
   37 to 39.9 (women)
b) 44 to 46.9 (men)
   40 to 41.9 (women)
c) 47 to 49.9 (men)
   42 to 44.9 (women)
d) 50 to 54.9 (men)
   45 to 47.9 (women)
e) above 54.9 or below 40 (men)
   above 47.9 or below 37 (women)

20. Uric acid (normal 3–5)
Is your uric acid level:
a) 4.0 or less
b) 4.1 to 4.9
c) 5.0 to 5.9
d) 6.0 to 6.9
e) 7.0 or more

21. Blood urea nitrogen (BUN) (normal 8–20)
Is your blood urea nitrogen:
a) less than 4
b) more than 4 but less than 6
c) more than 6 but less than 8
d) more than 8 but less than 10
e) more than 10 but less than 14
f) 14 or more but less than 16 (or more than 8 but less than 10)
g) 16 or more but less than 18

     h) 18 or more but less than 20
     i) 20 or more

22. Blood glucose (normal 80–120)
Is your blood glucose:
a) 91–104
b) 105–119 (or 81–90)
c) 120–127 (or 72–80)
d) 128–132 (or 67–71)
e) 133 or more (or 66 or less)

Reference points
The following measurements are a significant part of your medical history, but do not enter into the Supernutrition score. Record them each time that you record numbers 16–22.

23. Body temperature (normal 97.0–99.1)
24. Coagulation time (Lee-White) (normal 6–12 minutes)
25. Prothrombin time (Quick) (normal 10–15 seconds)

Total each column in Series III.
Give yourself 20 points for each *a* answer,
              15 points for each *b* answer,
              10 points for each *c* answer,
              5 points for each *d* answer and
              0 points for each *e–i* answer.
Enter your total at the bottom of the Scorecard. Maximum score for Series III is 140.

Total your scores for Series I, II, and III (maximum score is 500). Enter total on your Supernutrition Scoreboard (p. 279).

Multiply by 0.2 (or divide by 5) to obtain your Percentage of Relative Health.

See figure 32.5 for the interpretation of your score.

If You Can't Check with a Doctor

Of course, some of us do not have easy access to physicians or cannot afford visits to the doctor for the purposes of preventive medicine. This is unfortunate, but it is insufficient cause to prevent an effective measure of health improvement. If you are not under a doctor's care, you will have fewer facts and, therefore, your score will be less accurate than it could be. But a "modified" Supernutrition Score and "modified" Relative Health percentage can still be calculated. (See Figure 32.2.)

Without the information normally obtained in Series III and the surveillance of your family physician, be sure to look for danger signs such as extreme nervousness, eye whites turning yellow, unusual fatigue, unexplained diarrhea, irritability, heart palpitations, cloudy urine (not colored, but cloudy). Any of these symptoms may be due to lack of sleep, illness, excitement, overstimulation from too rapid an increase in vitamin or mineral intake, or a severe nutrient imbalance. Try cutting back on vitamin dosage for a three- or four-day period until the symptoms disappear. If they don't disappear in three or four days, see your physician. They are due to something else.

If you don't have a personal physician and are interested in locating a physician with a strong nutritional background, contact professional organizations such as the International Academy of Preventive Medicine, 10409 Town and Country Way, Suite 200, Houston, Texas 77024 (713–468–7851), or the American Academy of Medical Preventics at 9201 Sunset Boulevard, Suite 912, Los Angeles, California 90069 (213–278–0600)—or inquire at local health-food stores.

Reaching Your Supernutrition Point

An organized plan, not a prescription, the Supernutrition Program outlines a scientific procedure to reach *your* Supernutrition point, your own peak of health. Your guidance comes from your Supernutrition Score, not from me, from your physician, or from anyone else. As you exercise your right to alter your dietary intake constructively so that you reach your best health, your score will reflect your success or slippage.

The objective of the program is to reach your best health by regularly measuring your Supernutrition Score while systematically increasing your vitamin and mineral intake. The surest way to reach success is by a slow, steady, and safe progress. Start with a good foundation by having a blood-chemistry test and minor checkup by your family physician (an expensive and complete examination isn't needed, but it certainly won't hurt). The next step is to take your initial Supernutrition Score as previously explained. In choosing your starting levels of vitamins, you will find it convenient to select standard strengths that are commercially available. It is wise to start with low doses rather than high ones; step-by-step suggestions for gradually increasing your dosages of the various vitamins and minerals follow in the next section.

After two weeks on the program, you should measure your progress by taking your Supernutrition Score again. The amount of progress will depend on how good your health was to begin with, and how reliably you have followed the dosage suggestions.

If your starting health was near perfect, you will not see measurable progress for some time, but your health will progressively become optimized. On the other hand, if your initial health was far from ideal, your progress will be swifter and more noticeable right from the start. In the first two weeks you will notice dramatic improvements in energy, spirit, bowel regularity, and overall alertness. Instead of being weary, you will have drive; instead of dropping off to sleep at nine or ten, you will have the energy to exercise and see the late shows on TV if you wish.

Remember, supplements are to be used *in addition to* a balanced and varied diet of fresh, whole foods, *not in place of* those good foods. Never fall into the trap of believing you can eat junk as long as you take a vitamin pill.

There are many essential nutrients still to be discovered. Nutritionists know that unknown nutrients are in whole foods because experiments with purified synthetic diets of the known nutrients do not support life as well as natural diets.

The Value of Food Concentrates

Supernutrition is based on a diet of good foods, yet compensates for the fact that we do not always eat what we should. Our diet should be varied, balanced with the seven basic food groups, and consist primarily of whole, fresh, unprocessed foods whenever possible. We do not have to eat "organic" foods, but they will generally taste better (if fresh) and often be less contaminated by food additives or insecticides. If nutritional gaps occur in our food selection we can fill them with excellent food concentrates, such as wheat germ, desiccated liver, brewer's yeast, lecithin, yogurt, protein concentrates, etc.

A single capsule or tablet of a food concentrate taken daily is not going to make much difference in your health. (Only vitamin and mineral supplements are significantly effective in single-pill quantities.) There are, however, several reasons for taking food concentrates regularly in substantial quantities:

1) to add to your diet undiscovered nutrients the concentrates may contain;
2) to add known nutrients deficient in your normal diet (e.g., essential polyunsaturated fatty acids that occur in vegetable oils and nuts);
3) to add nutrients to balance a poor assortment of specific nutrients in your normal diet; and
4) to provide certain foods in a more acceptable form. (Those who dislike a particular food, for example, liver, usually have no objections to the taste of the concentrate.)

Generally, one or two tablespoons daily of each food concentrate will be helpful. The amounts recommended in Dr. Rinse's Breakfast (Chapter 31) are ideal for those with moderate heart disease. More would be even better, but be sure to consider calorie content and reduce the junk food in your diet by the *same* calorie amount.

A Few Words about Vitamin Selection

There are people who prefer not to take food concentrates. Their hope for balanced nutrition generally lies in vitamin and mineral supplements. Individual needs may vary from just a single multiple-vitamin pill each day to a variety of high-potency pills; the Supernutrition Program provides a guide to determining your needs.

The program suggests starting at a low dosage level and progressively increasing it. *Minimum* quantities are suggested for each step of the plan. Please note that these minimum quantities are not the actual amounts you *must* take; they are merely guidelines.

The formulations that you buy should contain *at least* the minimum amounts of each nutrient suggested. You will *not* find the exact formula suggested because each manufacturer provides a slightly different proportion of vitamins and nutrients. If the formulation you buy has at least the quantities suggested, it will work well. *If you can't find a formulation with the minimum quantities that I list, buy the one closest to it that you can.* As long as the minimums are met, you don't have to worry about "balance." Your body will take what is required and leave what is not needed, except in the cases of vitamins A and D, discussed below.

Several formulations are recommended in the Supernutrition Program: a "complete" vitamin-mineral formula, a "B-complex" formula, a "vitamin C" formula, a "vitamin E" formula, and a "mineral" formula. In combination, these formulas will allow you to select the right proportion of nutrients to fit your needs, without creating any imbalance.

Don't try to get by on the "complete" vitamin-mineral formula alone by taking several in order to reach the suggested minimum levels of the various vitamins. There are two important reasons for not doing this. First, you may take toxic amounts of vitamins A or D. Second, you will be stuck with the ratio of nutrients selected by a single manufacturer. Let your body judge what is best for you, not what is convenient or least expensive for a particular manufacturer.

You may discover that you do not tolerate a particular

formulation well. One may use an oil base that is wrong for you, causing an allergic reaction or indigestion. Another, instead of using niacinamide, may use niacin, which can cause "flushing" (reddening of the face). Change formulations if either is the case. Health-food store personnel can often help you to match formulations to your specific body tolerances.

You will find that you will get better results if you start with products of reliable quality. Once you have reached your highest Supernutrition Score, you can experiment with less expensive formulations, if you wish. But do not try to build health with vitamins or minerals of unreliable quality. It's much like putting cheap but inferior oil and gas in a car —it saves money today but causes expensive damage to-morrow.

Supernutrition Program

The Supernutrition Program is outlined below. Please note that, in all cases, the quantity of any vitamin listed is only a suggested one. The actual choices that you will make should depend on your needs and preferences.

Pregnant women should not attempt to find their Supernutrition point. And diabetics and those on anti-coagulant drugs should not begin the program except under their doctor's direct guidance.

1. Take your initial Supernutrition Score. (See pp. 280–281.)
2. *Start* your supplement program:
   a) 1 high-potency vitamin-mineral pill immediately after breakfast
   b) 2 B-complex tablets, one before or with breakfast, the other with the dinner meal
   c) 3 vitamin C tablets (250 mg each, preferably chewable), one with each meal
   d) 1 vitamin E capsule, 200 IU, at bedtime. (Start with 30 IU if you have high blood pressure. If diabetic, do not take vitamin E, except under your doctor's guidance.)
      Suggestions, not critical requirements, for steps *a* and

b are as follows. Additional information on vitamins is given in Appendix 9. You probably won't find these exact formulas; just select the ones close to the listed strength or higher in potency. These are suggested minimums.

Vitamins	Minimum Quantities
Vitamin A	10,000 USP
Vitamin D	400 USP
Vitamin B_1	10 mg
Vitamin B_2	10 mg
Vitamin B_6	5 mg
Vitamin B_{12}	4 mcg
Niacinamide (B_3)	50 mg
Pantothenic acid	10 mg
Choline	10 mg
Biotin	2 mcg
Folic acid	0.1 mg
Inositol	5 mg
Vitamin C	75 mg
Vitamin E	5 IU

Minerals	Minimum Quantities
Iodine	10 mcg
Manganese	1 mg
Magnesium	2 mg
Potassium	2 mg
Copper	1 mg
Zinc	1 mg
Iron	10 mg

Vitamin B Complex	Minimum Quantities
Vitamin B_1	10 mg
Vitamin B_2	10 mg
Vitamin B_6	10 mg
Vitamin B_{12}	4 mcg
Niacinamide (B_3)	10 mg
Pantothenic acid	20 mg
Other B-complex	
Choline	desirable
Biotin	desirable
Folic acid	desirable
Inositol	desirable

If you have heart disease, add with breakfast 50 mcg of selenium (organically bound in yeast) and 50 mg of vitamin B₁₅ (pangamic acid).

3. After two weeks, take your Supernutrition Score again, using the same values for Series III as you used when you took your initial Supernutrition Quiz.

4. Increase your supplements in accordance with the following schedule:
   a) 1 high-potency vitamin-mineral pill immediately after breakfast
   b) 3 B-complex tablets, one before or with breakfast, a second with dinner, and a third soon before bedtime
   c) 4 vitamin C tablets (250 mg each), one with each meal and one at bedtime
   d) 1 vitamin E capsule, 200 IU, at bedtime
   If you have heart disease, continue with breakfast 50 mcg of selenium and 50 mg of vitamin B₁₅.
   If dieting, pills should be taken 5 to 10 minutes before meals with a glass of water to help control hunger (by partially filling the stomach).

5. After two more weeks (one month total time since starting), take your third Supernutrition Score, again using the same values for Section III as you used in your first Supernutrition Quiz.

6. Increase your supplements to the following:
   a) 2 high-potency vitamin-mineral pills, one immediately after breakfast, another at bedtime
   b) 4 B-complex tablets, one before or with each meal plus a fourth at bedtime
   c) 6 vitamin C tablets (250 mg each), two with breakfast, one with lunch, two with dinner, and one at bedtime
   d) 2 vitamin E capsules (200 IU each), one with breakfast, one at bedtime
   If you have heart disease, continue with breakfast 50 mcg of selenium and 50 mg of vitamin B₁₅.

7. After two more weeks (six weeks after starting), take your fourth Supernutrition Score, again using the same values for Series III as you used in your first quiz.
   If your Supernutrition Score is lower than previous score (step 5), go back to step 4 and repeat steps 4, 5, 6, and 7

304 Supernutrition for Healthy Hearts

in proper sequence. If for the second time the score from step 7 is lower than step 5, step 4 is your optimum level.

If your Supernutrition Score is higher, then advance to step 8.

8. Increase your supplements to the following:
a) 2 high-potency vitamin-mineral pills, one immediately after breakfast, another with dinner
b) 5 B-complex tablets, two before or with breakfast, one before or with lunch, one with or near dinner, and two soon before bedtime
c) 2 vitamin C pills (1,000 mg each), one with breakfast, another with dinner
d) 3 vitamin E capsules (200 IU each), two with breakfast, another at bedtime
e) A mineral tablet at dinner or bedtime
A typical mineral tablet might contain the following:

Mineral	Minimum quantities
Calcium	125 mg
Magnesium	100 mg
Zinc	15 mg
Potassium	10 mg
Iodine	5 mcg
Manganese	1 mg
Copper	1 mg

It would be beneficial if the mineral tablet contains 200 USP of vitamin D and 100 mg of betaine hydrochloride.

If you have heart disease, continue with breakfast 50 mcg of selenium and increase your B_{15} to 75 mg.

If you are free of heart disease, add 15 mcg of selenium (organically bound in yeast) and 25 mg of vitamin B_{15} if your percentage of relative health is less than 93.

9. Take your fifth Supernutrition Score after two weeks (eight weeks after starting), again using the same values in Series III as you used in your first Supernutrition Quiz.

If your Supernutrition Score is lower than it was in step 7, go back to step 6 and repeat steps 6, 7, 8, and 9. If for the second time the score of step 9 is lower than that of step 7, step 6 is your optimum level.

If your Supernutrition Score is the same as in step 7, repeat steps 8 and 9.

If your Supernutrition Score is higher, advance to step 10.

10. Increase your supplements to the following:

    a) 2 high-potency vitamin-mineral pills, one immediately after breakfast, another with dinner

    b) 2 high-potency B-complex pills, one before or with breakfast, another soon before bedtime (or 8 regular B-complex pills). The high-potency B-complex tablet should have at least 50 mg of each of the major B vitamins.

    c) 3 vitamin C pills (1,000 mg each), one with breakfast, a second with dinner, a third at bedtime with a glass of milk

    d) 4 vitamin E capsules (200 IU each), 2 with breakfast, 2 at bedtime

    e) A mineral tablet at bedtime

    If you have heart disease, continue 50 mcg of selenium and increase your B_{15} to 100 mg.

    If you are free of heart disease, increase your selenium to 50 mcg and increase your B_{15} to 50 mg, if your percentage of relative health is less than 93.

11. The amounts in step 10 should bring most people to their Supernutrition point (highest score). Take your sixth Supernutrition Score after 2 weeks (10 weeks after starting) again using the same values for Series III as you used in your initial Supernutrition Quiz. Repeat the same pattern as in steps 5, 7, and 9, according to whether your Supernutrition Score is better, the same, or worse.

12. Maintain the same level of supplements as in steps 10 and 11.

13. After 2 weeks (12 weeks from the start), take your seventh Supernutrition Score. This time visit your doctor and get your second blood-chemistry and minor checkup.

14. Continue to adjust your supplement program, making variations only (plus or minus) in B-complex, B_{15} (pangamic acid), vitamin C, vitamin E, and mineral levels until you find your Supernutrition point—this will be the highest score achieved in periodically taking the quiz. Remember that many minerals (especially selenium) can be toxic, so don't overdo the suggested ranges on the labels. After vitamin and mineral levels are determined, you can experiment with other supplements such as lecithin, yeast, etc.

    Blood chemistries and minor checkups are suggested at
    —start
    —12 weeks

—9 months
—18 months
—once yearly after that

When your Supernutrition Score decreases, decrease dosage until an increase is seen or until it returns to the previous high. Be sure to increase the dose again to see if the decrease in score was real or a result of an unrelated event stemming from overwork, emotion, stress, illness, or whatever. You may not have sensed an illness because, rather than being sick in bed, you experienced only a decrease in energy. If the decrease in score appears again, decrease dosage—you have just passed your Supernutrition point. If the score increases, continue—you experienced an unrelated event or had a temporary response to the larger dose. Minimum variances in the score of less than 15 points may be disregarded.

The Supernutrition principle has built-in safety factors, both in terms of protecting your health and in preventing you from making mistakes or misinterpretations. The program includes "trend" and "repeat" principles to prevent false conclusions. If you are feeling good and your score is moving upward, it must be *sustained* or it is false and meaningless; if you are feeling good because of natural emotional cycles or psychological factors, you may get a sudden but temporary increase in your Supernutrition Score—this is a false peak and will disappear. A true Supernutrition peak follows a long upward trend and is sustained—within reasonable limits—at all times. A decrease might make you conclude that you have gone too high. The "repeat" principle requires you to confirm this by repeating the dosage. The plateau may occur at a point where your body has not learned to utilize beneficially the higher dose, but with time and continued improved health, the body *can* utilize that dose. The "repeat" may reveal that you have passed your plateau.

Don't be discouraged if you catch a cold three weeks after starting your program; it takes much longer to build up resistance. Also, unrelated events, such as a skin rash caused by a fung is, should not enter into the Supernutrition Score. Because not everything is known about nutrition and many of the changes are long-term, the Supernutrition Program is not perfect. But it is better than taking the RDA or taking vitamins haphazardly. It is the *best* program of vitamin sup- plementation *known today.*

An Unexpected Risk Indicator

An unexpected indicator has been determined that corre- lates with heart-disease incidence more reliably than any of the previously reported potential risk factors. It has an ad- vantage in that it is a physical sign that can be recognized by nearly anyone. A quick look at a friend or even yourself (if you can see your ears with the aid of a couple of mirrors) is all that is required to detect a high risk of heart disease.

If you don't have this telltale indicator, you can be reas- sured that even if you have chest pains, the odds are only one in ten that the pain is due to heart disease. Remember many pains such as indigestion, gas, nervousness, hiatal hernia, and the like, can cause chest pain.

However, if you do have this indicator, statistics suggest that if you also have chest pain, the odds shift to nine in ten that the pain is due to heart disease.

The problems in revealing the indicator is that people without it may not diligently follow the Total Protection Plan or give up smoking as they were planning to before they learned that they were not in a high-risk category. Those with the mark might feel doomed to heart disease, and give up efforts to protect themselves. If you see a family member or a friend with the mark, your attitude towards them may subconciously be affected. If you tell those with the mark about its significance, you may frighten the life out of them. Yet isn't this what has been done to a lesser degree with warnings concerning cholesterol level, smoking, and ele- vated blood pressure?

The difference is that when you are dealing with blood chemistry or blood pressure, you can see an improvement and thus have knowledge of your "improved" chances. The ear mark, however, may be irreversible and remain even after your vascular system improves. So even the presence of this mark does not necessarily indicate the present health of the individual.

What is this mark? Simply a deep diagonal crease in the earlobe as shown in figure 32.6. It begins at the lowest corner of the ear opening, then extends outward to the lobe. The mark is significant whether one or both ears are creased. Ear creases other than the type described are no cause for concern.

Remember, if you have the mark it does not mean that you are doomed, but it does mean that you should see your doctor and monitor the A, B, C, D, E, F factors of the Total Protection Plan. If you don't have the mark, it doesn't mean that you can ignore the Total Protection Plan either.

Figure 32.6 TELLTALE CREASE: The type of earlobe crease that indicates you're a likely heart attack victim begins at the lowest corner of the ear opening (arrow), then extends outward on the lobe in varying lengths. Other creases in the lobe are no cause for concern.

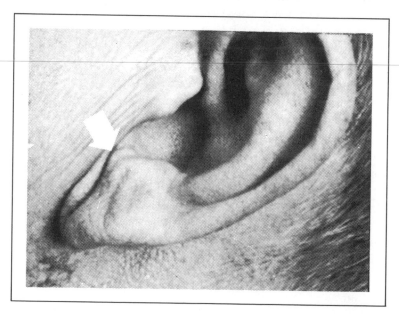

The crease is believed to be the result of atherosclerosis reducing the blood supply, thus causing the earlobe, which is composed of a large number of blood vessels, to contract or crease as a result of the diminished blood supply.

Dr. S. T. Frank was the first physician to report this aural clue of cardiovascular disease in 1973 (in the *New England Journal of Medicine*). Confirmations from follow-ups were published in 1974 and 1975.

In 1974, Dr. Edgar Lichstein and his colleagues (at the Division of Cardiology of the Mount Sinai School of Medicine in New York) reported on their observations of 531 heart patients: "The diagonal earlobe crease appears more commonly in patients with coronary heart disease and should be regarded as a coronary risk factor. Although other risk factors may be present in the same patient, this crease is easily noted and serves to identify this high-risk group. . . . In the group with coronary heart disease, the ear crease was present in 47 percent, diabetes mellitus in 16 percent, and hypertension in 29 percent." (*New England Journal of Medicine,* 1974)

In 1975, Dr. Jens Christiansen and his colleagues (at the Gentofte Hospital in Copenhagen, Denmark) stressed that the ear creases were not just a function of age. "The earlobe crease was more common in the patients with coronary heart disease than in the controls in the later decades [of life]. A higher correlation was found between coronary heart disease and the earlobe crease than between coronary heart disease and risk factors such as arterial hypertension, cigarette smoking, and diabetes mellitus. We agree that there is an increased prevalence of the diagonal earlobe crease with advancing age, but our results support the findings of Lichstein et al. that the presence of the earlobe crease is positively related to coronary heart disease." (*New England Journal of Medicine,* 1975)

At a 1974 American Heart Association meeting in Dallas, Dr. Jack Sternlieb of the Mayo Clinic reported, "According to our study of 121 coronary artery disease patients, a person with the crease who has coronary signs, such as pains in the chest, has about a 90 percent chance of having coronary artery disease. Of particular importance, however, is that the person who has symptoms of heart disease and does not have the earlobe crease has about a 90 percent chance of being *free* of coronary artery disease."

At this same 1974 American Heart Association meeting, Dr. Lichstein added, "I think the greatest significance of our research is for men between 45 and 60 [years of age]. If you have an earlobe crease and you are middle-aged, then you should be checked for other coronary risk factors."

In Summary

If you have heart disease, it should be comforting to know that you can make a total recovery and, in fact, be in better health than you have been in a decade or more.

Life is meant for living, so live all the days of your life. Preventing and curing heart disease is not only to add years to your life, but to add life to your years!

Do the best that you can to reduce the six controllable risk factors—A,B,C,D,E,F. Remember, it's

- A for Antioxidant nutrients (Chapters 9 through 14)
- B for Blood pressure (Chapters 22 and 23)
- C for cutting down on Cigarettes (Chapters 24 and 25)
- D for Diet—Calories do count (Chapter 26)
- E for Exercise (Chapters 27 and 28)
- F for Frustration—Get rid of most of it (Chapter 29)

The best years can lie ahead.

But do not become fanatical about one factor or another, because that could raise your frustration level.

Consider adding two other ingredients to the Total Protection Plan—love and faith. Each alone could accomplish miracles.

If you need assurance that the Total Protection Plan works, remember it has been 26 years (at this writing) since Dr. Rinse was "doomed" with heart disease. He is in better health today, enjoying life, and he has contributed much to his fellow man in that time.

Others, such as comedian Joey Bishop, have reported that their former heart problems "saved their lives." If you have a heart condition, it does not have to be the end of life; it can very well be a new beginning to a fuller, more enjoyable life.

It is never to late to change your habits. I have received hundreds of letters from people who had been sickly for decades until they changed their ways. In time, they regained their health and now feel better than they have in many years.

Begin now with the Total Protection Plan to make your heart five years younger in three months and ten years younger in nine months.

Appendix One
The Monoclonal-Proliferation Theory of Heart Disease Summarized

For many decades it was believed that cholesterol in food caused heart disease. Since 1965, a number of studies have shown that cholesterol does not cause heart disease, and that avoiding cholesterol or lowering blood cholesterol levels with polyunsaturates or drugs does not prevent heart disease. Since 1970, several American scientists have uncovered the origin of human atherosclerotic plaques, which cause clinical heart disease. A simplified explanation of the new theory of heart disease follows.

Arteries normally make cholesterol. Diseased arteries, however, make fibrous plaques which in turn produce excess cholesterol within the plaques. All cholesterol is produced from basic body chemicals in the cell, and is not dependent on the amount of cholesterol in the bloodstream or whether protein, fats, or carbohydrates are eaten.

The initial plaque formed by diseased arteries is due to a mutation of a cell in the artery wall. Certain chemicals in the bloodstream, including chemical pollutants, smoke components, and reactive molecular fragments called free radicals, cause a normal smooth muscle cell in the arterial wall to go haywire (mutate). The fibrous plaque consequently formed is essentially a benign tumor. Thus the origin of heart disease is akin to the origin of cancer.

The cell that mutated because of the presence of reactive chemicals reproduces itself (proliferates) in its new mutated form exactly, and all cells subsequently reproduced by this mutated parent cell are exact replicas (that is, they are monoclonal). They form a growth unique from normal arterial cells. This growth is the first step in plaque formation that has for years been missed by other researchers. Dr. Earl P. Benditt of the University of Washington made this discovery using sophisticated techniques of cell differentation with the electron microscope, coupled with chemical analyses of the enzymes present in each cell.

Monoclonal proliferation continues at a rate faster than normal cell growth, and cell crowding occurs. A second stage is reached in which the crowded cells produce collagen and cholesterol to form a fibrous mass. This second stage is the uncomplicated plaque that for years has been wrongly considered the first stage.

The third stage is a complication of the second stage, in which the fibrous mass has erupted through the arterial wall into the bloodstream. In this stage, calcium and cholesterol are attracted from the bloodstream and added to the fibrous mass by electrostatic-charge attraction. This complication adds to the plaque size and reduces blood flow, and also enhances blood clotting. However, even the third stage is independent of blood cholesterol level, for cholesterol would be attracted from the bloodstream regardless of the level of cholesterol in the blood.

Both stages one and three can be controlled by the Total Protection Plan outlined in the final chapter.

The monoclonal-proliferation theory is discussed from a more balanced point of view in a letter to me by Dr. Robert I. Levy, Director of the National Heart, Lung, and Blood Institute.

Thank you for your letter about the monoclonal aspect of the pathogenesis of atherosclerosis.

Certainly the Benditts' study has been a most imaginative and stimulating one. The basic observation that the raised fibrous or fibrofatty plaques are predominantly monoclonal appears to be firmly established by the work of the Benditts, by work from Heptinstall's laboratory at Johns Hopkins and by the work from

Thomas' laboratory at Albany. Such plaques are those typical of adult atherosclerosis and are generally regarded as mature, i.e. of considerable duration. Of course, technical matters have limited the observations to black females and only the aorta has been studied to date, so that, in a strict sense, one cannot speak of other vessels or of men.

However, there are additional observations to be added to the basic one of monoclonality. The work from Johns Hopkins also studied fatty streaks (mostly from older ages) and found that there was little evidence for monoclonality in such lesions. The Albany investigators attempted to relate monotypism to the thickness of lesions (see attached abstract from the November, 1976 Scientific Sessions of the American Heart Association). They found that thinner lesions were seldom monotypic while thicker lesions usually were.

The observations lend themselves to different interpretations. The Johns Hopkins laboratory has suggested that the data supports the view that the typical adult or mature plaques of atherosclerosis do not arise from fatty streak lesions. The origin of adult-type lesions from fatty streaks is itself a controversial issue and they view their data as possible evidence to the contrary. The Albany data, however, deals with plaques of adult type but of differing thickness and they suggest that this may indicate that plaques acquire monotypism gradually as they develop. That is, that monoclonality in plaques is acquired slowly by the preferential survival of a strain of cells rather than by the abrupt genetic transformation of a progenitor cell.

The question of genetic transformation versus genetic preferential survival or multiplication without transformation is central here, and it is probably fair to say that additional data will need to be obtained before the question can be resolved to everyone's satisfaction. That there are two profoundly different views of the pathogenesis of atherosclerosis is obvious, and they have profoundly different implications for the early or initial etiological events in the causation of plaques.

At the same time, we should not lose sight of the exciting finding that mature plaques are monoclonal. Their monotypism can be expected to have some influence on how uniformly a plaque will react to its environment of risk factors.

I hope these comments are helpful, and I thank you for your interest.

Sincerely yours,
Robert I. Levy
Director

Gina Kolata, reporter for *Science* magazine, discussed the new theory and has summarized the objections raised against the monoclonal-proliferation theory.

Although other investigators have confirmed the Benditts' results, several groups have recently raised objections to their interpretation. Philip Fialkow of the University of Washington, for example, points out that there is some evidence that plaques develop in layers. A group of cells may proliferate, then most die, and a few remaining cells proliferate again. If this is the case, a plaque could end up with cells of a single enzyme phenotype even though the plaque originated from many cells. Similarly, George Martin and his associates at the University of Washington School of Medicine argue that the Benditts' data do not necessarily indicate that plaques are formed by mutated or transformed cells. After studying a variety of cell lines, they discovered that cells that divide rapidly enjoy a selective advantage. Thus progeny of a single cell might take over a plaque that had a multicellular origin.

Somewhat different evidence against the monoclonal hypothesis is reported by Wilbur Thomas and his associates at Albany Medical College. These investigators found that plaques in swine are not monoclonal. They radioactively labelled the normal arterial tissue and induced lesions by feeding the animals diets high in cholesterol. If each lesion were formed from a single cell, the radioactivity of each lesion should be substantially less than the radioactivity of the surrounding cells of the artery. This did not occur. Instead the radioactivity of each lesion was not sufficiently diluted for it to be derived from one rather than many cells.

Thomas admits that the lesion in swine may not be analogous

to those of humans, but still maintains that the evidence advanced by the Benditts is not sufficient to support the monoclonal hypothesis. Despite these arguments against the monoclonal hypothesis, no one has yet succeeded in ruling it out. It, like the response-to-injury hypothesis, continues to have both supporters and detractors. Both hypotheses continue to suggest new experiments whose results, many believe, are narrowing the range of possible causes of and ways to prevent atherosclerosis. (*Science,* 1976.)

Secondary Plaques and Blood Cholesterol

The plaques caused by monoclonal proliferation are the primary plaques that cause clinical symptoms of cardiovascular disease. These plaques are a problem because of their fibrous nature. In addition to the monoclonal plaques, there are two other types of plaques: One type is due to injury of the arterial surface (endothelium) and is a less frequent cause of cardiovascular-disease symptoms. The other type is the "fatty streak" plaque which does not produce clinical symptoms and appears to do no damage.

Plaques appear to form most frequently near the junction of two arterial branches, as shown in Figures 3.1 through 3.5. This is in accordance with the physical laws of hemodynamics that predict that at arterial junctions blood flow is both turbulent and slowed near the vessel wall. Thus, near such junctions arterial surface damage can occur as blood platelets or other particles collide. And at such points, free radicals carried in the bloodstream can enter the arterial wall more easily because the surface blood flow is slower.

The free radicals entering the wall directly induce monoclonal-proliferation plaques, whereas the surface injury first causes platelets to adhere to the arterial wall at the injury site. Such adhered platelets are replaced by fibrous tissue within a few hours if the platelets are not broken up. (Discussed further in Chapter 9, on vitamin E). With time, the platelet-initiated plaque becomes difficult to differentiate from monoclonal plaques. Once either type forms near a junction, it enhances the effect of the junction (further slowing the flow of blood while increasing its turbulence) and accelerates plaque formation.

Plaques near junctions are especially subject to infiltration by lipoproteins because of the slower blood flow near the vessel wall. Several types of lipoproteins enter the wall easily, but only the low-density lipoprotein (LDL) is trapped and contributes to plaque building. Research is revealing that the blood levels of LDL may be a factor in accelerating the atherosclerotic process.

Incidentally, the blood levels of LDL determine how much cholesterol can be carried in the bloodstream before abnormalities occur. Thus a factor to monitor is *not* the blood level of cholesterol, but the *ratio* of blood cholesterol to blood LDL. A high cholesterol-to-LDL ratio may indicate a high probability for accelerated plaque growth (once plaque is formed). When the ratio is high, "free" cholesterol can be attracted to any plaque protruding through the wall. Note that the cholesterol-to-LDL ratio can be high even though the blood cholesterol level is low, depending of course on the availability of LDL.

Recent analysis of cholesterol levels in patients with heart disease has indicated that persons with low cholesterol levels in their high-density lipoproteins (HDL) may be at risk for heart disease. That is, in persons with any given level of LDL cholesterol, the probability of heart disease increases as the HDL cholesterol decreases. Conversely, high blood cholesterol levels, if the cholesterol is in the HDL, protects against heart disease.

Two mechanisms have been postulated to explain the role of HDL in the prevention of heart disease. The first mechanism by which HDL may prevent atherosclerosis is the apparent ability of HDL to remove cholesterol from the artery wall and to transport it to the liver for metabolism and removal from the body. An alternate possibility is that HDL may inhibit the uptake of LDL cholesterol by the artery wall.

The third type of plaque, the "fatty streak" plaque, occurs frequently, even in young babies. The fatty streaks contain no fiber and are reversible. Enzymes called lysosomes can remove cholesterol from fatty streaks. Fats can enter and leave fatty streaks readily. Fatty streaks occur in different patterns and have different composition. They are more similar to the marbled streaks of fat in steak, whereas the monoclonal plaques are more similar to gristle.

In summary, the plaques that cause heart disease are fibrous in nature before accumulating cholesterol and are not related to fat or cholesterol in the diet. These plaques, of monoclonal origin, can be initiated by free radicals from cigarette smoke, high blood pressure, chemical pollution, chlorine (not chloride), stress, hypoxia (shortage of oxygen in the artery wall), and the like.

The plaques formed as a result of arterial surface injury are a relatively minor cause of clinical symptoms, but can be accelerated to become serious when the cholesterol-to-LDL ratio is high. And finally, the fatty streaks, much like harmless fat deposits, occur in the young and healthy, and have not been shown to be related to clinical symptoms of heart disease.

The establishment of elevated LDL and lowered HDL as independent risk factors for the development of atherosclerosis now necessitates determination of these cholesterol fractions individually. Merely measuring total blood cholesterol is no longer an acceptable index of the risk of developing heart disease. These cholesterol fractions are in no way related to the cholesterol in the diet in normal people, but do have genetic and nutritive involvement.

Appendix Three
Free Radicals Explained

A free radical is an atom or group of atoms possessing an odd (unpaired) electron. Most free radicals are extremely reactive because of their tendency to gain (capture) an additional electron and thus be complete. When a free radical is formed, energy is supplied to the fragment during its cleavage from the parent molecule, and this energy-rich fragment tends strongly to lose energy by the formation of a new chemical bond. Free-radical reactions generally initiate chain reactions, producing more free radicals and reacted products. One free radical can produce chain reactions altering thousands and thousands of molecules.

A free radical is not to be confused with a charged ion. A free radical can be thought of as an unsaturated complex. Most free radicals persist for only a few thousandths of seconds, but stable free radicals such as triphenylmethyl and 2.2-diphenyl-1-picrylhydrazyl can be stored in a bottle. A free radical can be detected by paramagnetic resonance and phosphorescence because of its unpaired electron.

Appendix Four
Dietary Restrictions for Hyperlipoproteinemia

(Suggested by the Office of Heart Information, National Heart, Lung, and Blood Institute)

Type	Diet
I	Low fat (less than 25g/day), supplemented with medium chain triglycerides High carbohydrate
II	Low cholesterol (less than 300 mg/day) Low saturated fat, supplemented with unsaturated fat. (Weight reduction has little effect except in type IIb)
III	Weight reduction to ideal body weight Low cholesterol (less than 300 mg/day) Balanced diet (40% fat, 40% carbohydrate) Low alcohol intake
IV	Weight reduction to ideal body weight Low carbohydrate (100–150 g/day) if cholesterol remains elevated Low alcohol intake
V	Weight reduction to ideal body weight High protein Modest fat and carbohydrate reduction Low alcohol intake

Appendix Five
An Indication That Vitamin E Prevents Heart Disease

A survey I conducted of nearly twenty thousand vitamin E users produced an unexpected result. It was found that the amount of heart disease in any age group decreased proportionally with the length of time of taking vitamin E. A summary of this statistical survey and its interpretation is given in Chapter 10. The data on which those conclusions are based are presented here. The questionnaire used in the survey was published in the August 1974 issue of *Prevention* magazine, and detailed reports were published in the January through August 1976 issues of *Prevention*. *Prevention*'s cooperation in conducting this survey is greatly appreciated.

Table A5.1

Survey Respondents

Age Group	Number in Group	Number with Heart Disease
90–99	106	7
80–89	1,064	284
70–79	4,060	1,073
60–69	6,459	1,543
50–59	6,205	818
	17,894	3,725

Table A5.2

Heart Disease Incidence in Vitamin E Users Aged 50–59

Years Taking Vitamin E	Number in Group	Survey Participants with Heart Disease Developed Prior to Taking Vitamin E						Survey Participants with Insufficient Data to Classify Heart Disease as Prior or Not						Survey Participants with Heart Disease Developed While Taking Vitamin E						Survey Participants Free of Heart Disease	
		Better #	%	Same #	%	Worse #	%	Better #	%	Same #	%	Worse #	%	Better #	%	Same #	%	Worse #	%	#	%
30+	24	0		0		0		0		0		0		0		0		0		24	100
25–29	18	0		0		0		0		0		0		0		0		0		18	100
20–24	116	4	3.4	0		0		0		0		0		0		0		0		112	96.6
15–19	228	14	6.1	2	0.9	0		4	1.8	2	0.9	0		0		0		0		206	90.4
10–14	405	36	8.9	2	0.5	0		5	1.2	1	0.2	0		1	0.2	0		0		360	88.9
6–9	690	73	10.6	6	0.9	1	0.1	8	1.2	1	0.1	1	0.1	1	0.1	1	0.1	0		598	86.7
4–5	1407	141	10.0	28	2.0	7	0.5	9	0.6	1	0.1	2	0.1	5	0.4	1	0	1	0.1	1213	86.2
1–3	2887	276	9.6	62	2.1	11	0.4	22	0.8	4	0.1	6	0.2	7	0.2	8	0.3	6	0.2	2485	86.1
less than 1	269	25	9.3	3	1.1	8	3.0	0		0		0		0		0		0		233	86.6
Subtotal	6044																			5249	86.8
0	161																			138	85.7
Total	6205																			5387	86.8

Spearman-Rho Stat Rho is 0.92.

The percentages listed in the chart refer to the members of each group of "years taking vitamin E" applying to each category listed above. In Table A5.2, as an example, 3.4 percent of those taking vitamin E for 20–24 years and had prior heart disease report their heart disease better; this indicates that of the 116 respondents, 4 had prior heart disease (3.4 percent of the group) and all 4 were helped appreciably by vitamin E. Thus of the 3.4 percent of the responding group with prior heart disease, 100 percent were helped by vitamin E.

Heart Disease Incidence in Vitamin E Users Aged 60–69

Years Taking Vitamin E	Number in Group	Survey Participants with Heart Disease Developed Prior to Taking Vitamin E						Survey Participants with Insufficient Data to Classify Heart Disease as Prior or Not						Survey Participants with Heart Disease Developed While Taking Vitamin E						Survey Participants Free of Heart Disease	
		Better #	%	Same #	%	Worse #	%	Better #	%	Same #	%	Worse #	%	Better #	%	Same #	%	Worse #	%	#	%
30+	29	0	0	0		0	0	0		0		0		0		0		0		29	100
25–29	33	2	6.1	1	3.0	0	0	0		0		0		0		0		0		30	90.9
20–24	148	11	7.4	3	2.0	0	0	2	1.4	0		0		3	2.0	0		0		127	85.8
15–19	352	29	8.2	9	2.6	0	0	2	0.6	1	0.3	0		5	1.4	0		0		306	86.9
10–14	779	99	12.7	17	2.2	1	0.1	3	0.4	0		0		5	0.6	0		0		654	84.0
6–9	811	142	17.5	22	2.7	3	0.4	1	0.1	1	0.1	0		3	0.4	0		1	0.1	638	79.0
4–5	1372	283	20.6	48	3.5	6	0.4	1	0.1	0		0		5	0.4	0		1	0.1	1028	74.9
1–3	2487	476	19.1	91	3.7	29	1.2	37	1.5	8	0.3	6	0.2	6	0.2	8	0.3	11	0.4	1815	73.0
less than 1	247	58	23.5	12	4.9	5	2.0	0	0	0		0	0	0	0	8	0.1	0	0	172	69.6
Subtotal	6258	1100	17.6	203	3.2	44	0.7	46	0.8	10	0.1	6	0.1	27	0.4	8	0.1	13	0.2	4799	76.9
0	171																			117	68.4
TOTAL	6459																			4916	76.1

Spearman-Rho Stat: Rho is 0.94

The percentages listed in the chart refer to the members of each group of "years taking vitamin E" applying to each category listed above. In Table A5.3, as an example, 6.1 percent of those taking vitamin E for 25–29 years report their heart disease better; this indicates that of the 33 respondents, 3 had prior heart disease (9.1 percent of the group) and 2 were helped appreciably by vitamin E. Thus of the 9.1 percent of the responding group with prior heart disease, 66 percent were helped by vitamin E.

Heart Disease Incidence in Vitamin E Users Aged 70–79

Years Taking Vitamin E	Number in Group	Survey Participants with Heart Disease Developed Prior to Taking Vitamin E						Survey Participants with Insufficient Data to Classify Heart Disease as Prior or Not						Survey Participants with Heart Disease Developed While Taking Vitamin E						Survey Participants Free of Heart Disease	
		Better #	%	Same #	%	Worse #	%	Better #	%	Same #	%	Worse #	%	Better #	%	Same #	%	Worse #	%	#	%
30+	96	6	6.3	0	0	0	0	1	1.0	0	0	0	0	4	4.2	0	0	0	0	85	88.5
20–29	268	38	14.2	2	0.7	0	0	6	2.2	2	0.7	0	0	0	0	1	0.4	0	0	219	81.8
10–19	862	132	15.3	11	1.3	2	0.2	4	0.5	2	0.2	1	0.1	2	0.2	0	0	0	0	708	82.1
6–9	567	138	24.3	24	4.2	2	0.4	0	0	0	0	0	0	2	0.4	0	0	0	0	401	70.7
4–5	713	172	24.1	28	3.9	3	0.4	0	0	0	0	0	0	3	0.4	1	0	1	0.1	506	71.0
1–3	1340	337	25.1	62	4.2	14	1.0	0	0	0	0	0	0	0	0	1	0.1	0	0	926	69.1
less than 1	96	22	22.9	4	4.2	8	8.3	0	0	0	0	0	0	0	0	0	0	0	0	62	64.6
Subtotal	3942	845	21.4	131	3.3	29	0.7	11	0.3	4	0.1	1	0.0	11	0.3	2	0.05	1	0.0	2907	73.7
0	113																			80	67.8
TOTAL	4030																			2987	73.6

Spearman-Rho Stat: Rho is 0.96

The percentages listed in the chart refer to the members of each group of "years taking vitamin E" applying to each category listed above. In Table A5.4, as an example, 6.3 percent of those taking vitamin E for 30 years or more had prior heart disease, and all report their heart disease better; this indicates that of the 96 respondents, 6 had prior heart disease (6.3 percent of the group) and all 6 were helped appreciably by vitamin E. Thus of the 6.3 percent of the responding group with prior heart disease, 100 percent were helped by Vitamin E.

Heart Disease Incidence in Vitamin E Users Aged 80–89

Years Taking Vitamin E	Number in Group	Survey Participants Heart Disease Developed Prior to Taking Vitamin E						Survey Participants with Heart Disease Developed While Taking Vitamin E		Survey Participants Free of Heart Disease	
		Better		Same		Worse					
		#	%	#	%	#	%	#	%	#	%
30+	6*	0	0	0	0	0	0	0**	0**	6	100
20–29	104	15	14.4	0	0	0	0	0**	0**	89	85.6
10–19	266	48	18.0	0	0	0	0	2	0.8	216	81.2
6–9	136	43	31.6	1	0.7	0	0	(1)**	(0.7)	91	66.9
4–5	200	52	26	8	4.0	4	2.0	(1)**	(0.5)	135	67.5
1–3	274	67	24.5	11	4.0	6	2.2	0	0	190	69.3
less than 1	32*	6	18.8	2	6.3	1	3.1	0	0	23	71.8
Subtotal	1018	231	22.7	22	2.1	11	1.1	(4)*	(0.4)	750	73.7
0	46*	—	—	—	—	—	—	—	—	30	65.2***
Total	1064	—	—	—	—	—	—	—	—	780	73.3

*Sample group size insignificant

**No confirmed cases

***Higher than normal due to proper diet and multivitamins

Spearman-Rho Stat: Rho is 0.92

The percentages listed in the chart refer to the members of each group of "years taking vitamin E" applying to each category listed above. In Table A5.5, as an example, 14.4 percent of those taking vitamin E for 20–29 years report their heart disease better; this indicates that of the 104 respondents, 15 had prior heart disease (14.4 percent of the group) and all 15 were helped appreciably by vitamin E. Thus of the 14.4 percent of the responding group with prior heart disease, 100 percent were helped by vitamin E.

Heart Disease Incidence in Vitamin E Users Aged 90–99

Years Taking Vitamin E	Number in Group	Survey Participants Heart Disease Developed Prior to Taking Vitamin E						Survey Participants with Heart Disease Developed While Taking Vitamin E		Survey Participants Free of Heart Disease	
		Better		Same		Worse					
		#	%	#	%	#	%	#	%	#	%
30+	3	0	0	0	0	0	0	0	0	3	100
20–29	0	0	0	0	0	0	0	0	0	0	0
10–19	31	1	3.2	0	0	0	0	0	0	29	96.8
6–9	12	1	8.3	0	0	0	0	0	0	11	91.7
4–5	9	1	11.1	0	0	0	0	1	11.1	7	77.8
1–3	38	1	2.6	1	2.6	0	0	0	0	36	94.8
less than 1	5	0	0	0	0	0	0	0	0	5	100
Subtotal	98	4	4.1	1	1.0	0	0	1	1.0	92	93.9
0	8	—	—	1	12.5	0	0	—	—	7	87.5
TOTAL	106	4	3.8	2	1.9	0	0	1	0.9	99	93.4

Spearman-Rho Stat: not applied because of small sample size

The percentages listed in the chart refer to the members of each group of "years taking vitamin E" applying to each category listed above. In Table A5.6, as an example, percent of those taking vitamin E for 10–19 years report their heart disease better; this indicates that of the 31 respondents, 1 had prior heart disease (3.2 percent of the group) and that individual was helped appreciably by vitamin E. Thus of the 3.2 percent of the responding group with prior heart disease, 100 percent were helped by vitamin E.

Appendix Six
Reviving a Stopped Heart
with Cardiopulmonary Resuscitation

As pointed out in Chapter 1, a large portion of the decrease in heart-attack deaths has been due to the new technology in emergency care. The increased use of paramedics and mobile intensive-care ambulances deserves most of the credit. Still more lives can be saved, for there is one emergency technique used by paramedics and physicians alike to revive stopped hearts that can be learned even by those without paramedical training. This technique, called CPR (cardiopulmonary resuscitation), can save 50,000 lives a year if it is known by enough people and applied within three minutes of heart stoppage. CPR is the technique used by firemen to revive victims overcome by smoke. In Seattle, Washington, over 100,000 citizens have been trained in CPR, and already the heart-attack survival rate has climbed from 12 percent to 20 percent.

If CPR is started within one minute of a heart attack, the chance of recovery is 98 percent. If CPR is delayed by four minutes, the chance of recovery is 50 percent. If there is a seven-minute delay, the victim has only an 8 percent chance. More than 45 percent of the individuals resuscitated (after heart attack, suffocation by smoke, or drowning) make complete recovery.

Training requires less than three hours and classes are taught regularly at local American Red Cross chapters, municipal fire departments, and neighborhood Y's. A brief summary is given here to show you how easy the technique is and to serve as a reminder after you have received the training.

CPR consists of three basic steps as simple as ABC:

A — Air passageway opened by head-tilt method
B — Breathing restored by mouth-to-mouth breathing
C — Circulation restored by external heart compression

The details of CPR are:

A. Tilt the head back to open the air passageway.
B. 1. Determine If the victim is breathing by watching or touching the chest, listening for breaths, or feeling the breath on your cheek.
2. If the victim is not breathing, blow your breath into the victim's mouth to inflate the lungs. Your lips must form a seal with the victim's lips, and the victim's nostrils must be pinched closed. If the technique is done properly, the victim's chest will rise when you blow into the mouth. Give four quick, full breaths.
3. If the chest didn't rise, check the throat for a blockage and remove any foreign matter with your fingers. If no blockage is found, check head tilt and seals. Give four more quick, full breaths.
C. 1. Determine if the victim has a pulse by feeling the carotid arteries on each side of the windpipe.
2. If you can detect no pulse, compress the chest by pushing down on the sternum (breastbone) at two finger spaces above its tip (lower end). The chest should be compressed 1.5 to 2 inches with the heel of the hand.
3. Alternately give 15 compressions at the rate of about 80 per minute, and 2 quick, full lung inflations.
4. Repeat until victim is revived or professional help arrives.

Appendix Seven
Tasty Variations on a Health Theme by Dr. Rinse*

A quarter of a century ago, when he was 51, physical chemist Jacobus Rinse, Ph.D., suffered what his doctors told him was a heart attack. Subsequently, he was plagued by angina pains and the prognosis was that if he took good care of himself, he might live another 10 years.

Last winter, at the age of 76, Dr. Rinse took advantage of the snow that blanketed Vermont to start a new hobby—skiing.

He attributes his current health and vitality to a nutritional program based on a "mash" consisting of granular soybean lecithin, debittered brewer's yeast, raw wheat germ, bone meal and polyunsaturated oil. In addition, he takes vitamin C, vitamin E and often eats other healthful foods such as bran, yogurt and fruit.

Late last year, we published two articles by Dr. Rinse on his personal experiences, which concluded with his instructions for making what other people now call the "Rinse Breakfast Mash." Many people, we discovered, were anxious to use this formula, but some ran into problems with the taste, while others complained that they didn't like to eat cereal for breakfast every morning. So we put our Fitness House staff to work incorporating the basic ingredients of the mash into a variety of recipes that can be served at breakfast, lunch or supper. And frankly, we were amazed at the delicious results!

*Prevention, April 1976.

First, for the benefit of those who did not read Dr. Rinse's articles, the basic ingredients are one tablespoon each of granular lecithin, debittered brewer's yeast and raw wheat germ, with one *teaspoon* of bone meal. To two tablespoons of the above mixture, add one tablespoon or less of dark brown sugar, one tablespoon of safflower or other polyunsaturated oil and enough milk to dissolve the sugar and yeast. Finally, either add some yogurt to increase the consistency, and eat as is, or add the mixture to some cold or hot cereal.

Dr. Rinse's Pancakes

Many people enjoy a plate of pancakes for breakfast, and we found that adding the basic Rinse formula—lecithin, debittered brewer's yeast, wheat germ and bone meal—didn't bother the good taste a bit.

¾	cup whole wheat pastry flour
4	tablespoons Dr. Rinse's formula
½	teaspoon salt
1–2	tablespoons brown sugar
½	teaspoon baking powder
1	egg (optional)
1	tablespoon safflower oil
½	cup skim milk
1	tablespoon safflower oil (for pan)

Measure whole wheat pastry flour, Dr. Rinse's formula, salt and brown sugar. Beat an egg and add oil and milk to the egg. Add egg mixture to the dry mixture. If a thinner pancake is desired, omit the egg or add more milk.

Brown pancakes in the second tablespoon of safflower oil. Add more oil if necessary.

Serves two (two 4-inch pancakes each).

Wheatless Granola and Dr. Rinse's Formula

Granola is one of those foods that is associated with breakfast, but which is really adaptable to any meal. For those of us who are addicted to between-meal snacks, granola can be a boon—supplying nourishment as well as lots of satisfying *chewing*. With Dr. Rinse's Mash added, we enjoy still another benefit.

1 ½   cups rolled oats
½   cup rolled rye
½   cup bran
½   cup ground almonds
½   cup sunflower seeds
½   cup unsweetened coconut
2   tablespoons honey
2   tablespoons oil
¼   cup water

Combine above ingredients, stirring until grains and nuts are well coated. Pour the mixture into a large, shallow baking pan which has been lightly oiled and toast in a low oven (250°) for 1 ½ hours, stirring every 10 to 15 minutes or until mixture is dry and lightly browned and crisp. Remove cereal from the oven and allow it to cool. Store in glass jar in refrigerator.

To use, take:

½   cup granola
2   tablespoons Dr. Rinse's mixture
1   tablespoon safflower oil

Add milk, yogurt or sugar to taste.

Dr. Rinse's Omelet

If you asked the first three people you ran into what meal they usually associate with omelets, you'd probably get three different answers. Omelets are good for breakfast, good for lunch, good for a light supper. And with Dr. Rinse's Mash included, they're even better.

2   eggs
2   tablespoons Dr. Rinse's formula
¼   cup milk
1   tablespoon safflower oil

Beat eggs and add formula and milk. Warm oil in pan and pour in egg mixture. When egg begins to solidify, lift up egg with fork and allow liquid to run underneath to cook. Fold over and turn out onto serving plate. Serve immediately. Cheese, sautéed mushrooms, or chopped tomatoes could be placed inside the omelet before folding over. Serves one.

Every now and then, it's nice just to spread something good on a slice of whole grain bread. There's nothing better than Dr. Rinse's Mash. And for this, the Fitness House staff came up with not one but *two* variations.

Spread #1

2 tablespoons Rinse formula
1 tablespoon safflower oil
1 tablespoon brown sugar
1 tablespoon peanut butter
2 teaspoons boiling water

Mix the above ingredients and spread on a slice of bread.

Spread #2

2 tablespoons Rinse formula
1 tablespoon dark brown sugar
1 tablespoon safflower oil
2 tablespoons peanut butter
2 tablespoons rolled oats

Mix above ingredients and spread on bread.

Jane Kinderlehrer's Bran Muffins à la Dr. Rinse

1 cup whole wheat flour
1½ cups coarse bran
3 tablespoons wheat germ
3 tablespoons lecithin granules
3 tablespoons nutritional yeast
3 teaspoons bone meal powder
1 teaspoon baking soda
½ teaspoon grated orange rind
½ teaspoon cinnamon
¼ teaspoon cloves
few gratings of nutmeg
1 egg

⅓ cup blackstrap molasses
½ cup raisins soaked in ¾ cup hot water
½ cup sunflower seeds or chopped walnuts

Combine all the dry ingredients. Beat the egg with the liquid from the raisins and add the blackstrap molasses to this mixture. Combine the two mixtures. Add the raisins and the sunflower seeds or walnuts. Bake in buttered muffin tins for 20 minutes at 350°.

Yield: one dozen muffins.

Nutrients That Protect against Heart Disease and Their Specific Functions

VITAMINS

vitamin B_3	—lowers blood cholesterol level
source	—Brewer's yeast, meats, poultry, fish, peanuts, whole grains
vitamin B_6	—normalizes sugar and fat metabolism
	—required for lecithin synthesis
source	—meats, whole grains, organ meats, Brewer's yeast, legumes, green leafy vegetables
vitamin B_{13}	—strengthens heart
	—speeds recovery from heart attack
source	—root vegetables, seeds, whey
vitamin B_{15}	—increases available oxygen
	—decreases need for oxygen
	—lowers arterial pressure
	—enhances the circulatory blood volume
	—normalizes potassium and sodium balance
	—speeds recovery from heart attack
	—stimulates protein metabolism to repair heart damage
	—suppresses heart pain
	—normalizes fat transport
	—lowers blood cholesterol level
	—lessens area of damage during a heart attack
source	—Brewer's yeast, seeds, liver, rice, whole grains

choline	—required to make lecithin
source	—egg yolks, organ meats, Brewer's yeast, whole grains, lecithin
vitamin C	—removes plaque from artery walls
	—lowers blood cholesterol
	—needed for protection against stress
	—helps potentiate vitamin E
	—maintains proper arterial and capillary permeability
source	—citrus fruits, sprouted seeds, tomatoes
vitamin E	—normalizes blood-platelet adhesion (blood stickiness)
	—antioxidant action prevents monoclonal proliferation
	—prevents clots and dissolves existing clots
	—improves oxygen transportation by red blood cells
	—aids energy transfer in the heart, making the heart more efficient in oxygen usage; reduces oxygen consumption
	—prevents undesirable scarring of heart disease, while promoting a strong patch scar after an infarction
	—improves capillary permeability
	—often normalizes blood pressure
	—is a capillary vasodilator
	—reduces need for nitroglycerin in angina patients
	—reduces need for anticoagulants in heart patients
	—protects against excess polyunsaturates
	—survey results indicate a role in preventing heart disease
source	—whole grains, eggs, vegetable oils, leafy vegetables, organ meats

MINERALS

calcium	—required for heart contraction
	—reduces body lead content, thus protecting against a cause of high blood pressure

source	—milk and milk products, green leafy vegetables
chromium	—required for sugar and fat metabolism
source	—whole grains, Brewer's yeast, clams
magnesium	—required for heart-muscle relaxation (so that the heart contracts again for the next beat) —lowers blood pressure —required for proper potassium retention —required to make lecithin
source	—whole grains, nuts, green leafy vegetables, egg yolks
potassium	—required to maintain heartbeat regularity
source	—parsley, bananas, prunes, tomatoes, raisins, oranges, seeds, whole grains
selenium	—required to properly utilize vitamin E —normalizes blood pressure (prostaglandins) —detoxifies cadmium (which raises blood pressure) —reduces monoclonal proliferation —required for coenzyme Q production —reduces angina pain
source	—eggs, whole grains, garlic, onions, Brewer's yeast, tuna
zinc	—reduces body cadmium content —promotes healing of heart-tissue damage
source	—seeds, seafood, organ meats, Brewer's yeast

FOOD SUPPLEMENTS

lecithin	—lowers blood cholesterol level —provides essential polyunsaturates —normalizes fat transport —required for artery cell-membrane health —required for prostaglandin regulation
source	—egg yolk, soybeans, corn
fibers (bran, alfalfa, etc.)	—reduce blood cholesterol level
source	—whole grains, celery, bran, alfalfa, fruit

garlic   —reduces plaque formation
                      —lowers blood pressure
                      —normalizes blood-platelet adhesion

yogurt   —lowers blood cholesterol level

Vitamin Guide with Supernutrition Curves

To guide you in maximizing your Supernutrition Score and optimizing your health, use the discussions, suggestions, and Supernutrition curves in the following section. Each critical nutrient is discussed separately, and a guide is provided to show you relative relationships between the RDA, optimum intake, and toxicity diseases.

The Supernutrition curve illustrates the relationship between health and nutrient intake. The horizontal axis represents nutrient intake, with greatest amounts on the right; the vertical scale represents health, the best being at the top. The object is to optimize your health—to find the nutrient level that gives you the highest Supernutrition Score, which is the peak at point *D* on the curve. This is called the Supernutrition point. Point 4, directly below the Supernutrition point on the straight line *BE,* represents the amount of nutrients that you should take for best health. Point 1 is the official RDA, point 2 is a typical Supernutrition starting point, point 3 is the point at which one generally begins to feel the effects of the program, and point 5 is the level at which toxic effects begin to show in some people. Point 6 is a dangerously toxic level.

You now have the facts to help you find your best health —a *superior* health. The Supernutrition Score will tell you how well you are doing, and the Supernutrition curve will tell you what you need to know about each vitamin as you improve your health.

This is a start. The information is here for you to construct your supplement plan; suggestions (not prescriptions) are offered, and facts about the use of Supernutrition are given. The rest is up to you. Do not become a fanatic or a "health nut," but *do* read all you can to learn more about how nutrition affects your health; it is a good idea to subscribe to one or two nutrition magazines. A few of the more popular magazines available in the United States are listed on page 371 for your convenience.

The Supernutrition Curves

Vitamin A (Retinal or Retinol), Provitamin A (Carotene)

Vitamin A is a fat-soluble vitamin with known toxicity. Although its toxicity has been exaggerated, it is a factor well worth consideration. Carotene is converted in the body to vitamin A (retinol); it comes from vegetable sources (carrots, peas, lettuce, sweet potatoes, and tomatoes). Retinol comes from animal sources (liver, eggs, and dairy foods).

Agreed function: Vitamin A is necessary to normal growth and to skeletal development. It is also important in maintaining the health of the cells of mucous membranes and skin and in the normal functioning of all tissue. It is essential to the regeneration of visual purple in the eye and thus especially critical to night vision.

Speculative function: There are legitimate signs that vitamin A is essential to tissue health, especially in preventing precancerous cells from becoming cancerous. Similar evidence indicates that vitamin A plays a role in the prevention of colds and other viral infections.

Deficiency signs: Gross deficiency of vitamin A causes night blindness (nyctalopia); dry, rough skin; and a thickening of the cornea of the eye (xerophthalmia), which may lead to ulceration and blindness.

Toxicity signs: Dry, rough skin, yellowing of skin and eye whites, painful joint swellings, and nausea.

Precautions: None known.

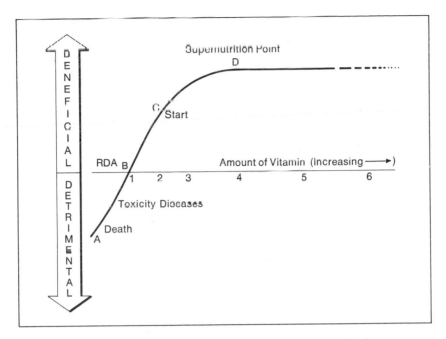

Figure A9.1 Supernutrition Curve: Vitamin A

Typical values

Points	Value
1.	RDA is 5,000 IU.
2.	Supernutrition starting point is 10,000 IU.
3.	20,000 IU.
4.	25,000 IU to 35,000 IU.
5.	75,000 IU.
6.	200,000 IU.

Preferred forms: (1) mixture of vitamin A (retinol) palmi-nate plus carotene; (2) vitamin A (retinol) palminate; (3) fish oils; and (4) carotene (vegetable oils).

Dosage advice: Absorbed best if taken with meals.

Vitamin B₁ (Thiamine)

Thiamine is a water-soluble vitamin with no known toxic effects if taken with other members of the vitamin B complex. Good sources are meat, fish, poultry, eggs, whole-grain breads, and cereals.

Agreed function: Thiamine is essential to appetite and to enable the body to use sugars and other carbohydrates. It is also necessary for the proper functioning of the nervous system.

Speculative function: To correct certain enzyme deficiencies and improve mental processes.

Figure A9.2 Supernutrition Curve: Vitamin B₁

Typical values

Points	Values
1.	RDA is 1.5 mg.
2.	Supernutrition starting point is 10–25 mg.
3.	50 mg.
4.	100 mg.
5.	Does not apply.
6.	Does not apply.

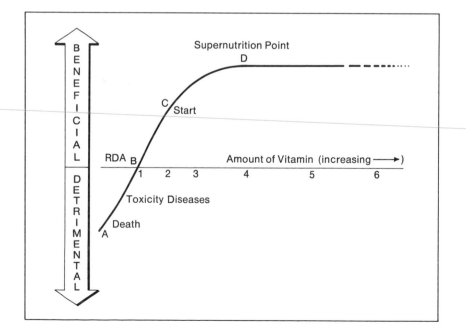

Deficiency signs: Fatigue, insomnia, irritability, loss of appetite, irregularity. Also heart and circulatory disturbances, digestive disturbances, muscle tenderness, weight loss, neuritic pain, forgetfulness, lassitude, mental inadequacy. Gross deficiency results in beriberi, a fatal heart disease among other things.

Toxicity signs: None known when taken orally. Repeated injections have occasionally caused sensitization. Colors the urine yellow but this is normal.

Precautions: Take with all major B-complex vitamins. Reduce dosage if heart palpitations occur.

Preferred forms: None.

Dosage advice: Take in divided doses 2 to 4 times a day (exact times not critical). Water-soluble vitamins, such as this member of the B complex, are quickly removed from the body by the kidneys.

Vitamin B₂ (Riboflavin)

Riboflavin is a water-soluble vitamin with no known toxic effects if taken with other members of the vitamin B complex. Good sources are milk, cheese, ice cream, liver, fish, poultry, eggs, and whole-grain breads and cereals.

Agreed function: Riboflavin is necessary in the oxidative process of metabolism.

Speculative function: To correct certain enzyme deficiencies and improve mental processes.

Deficiency signs: Riboflavin deficiency produces mouth irritation, dry scaling of the red surface of the lips and corners of the mouth, magenta-colored tongue, dermatitis, abnormal intolerance of the eyes to light, the release of tears, and eye redness.

Toxicity signs: None known.

Precautions: Take with all major B-complex vitamins. Reduce dosage if heart palpitations occur.

Preferred forms: None.

Dosage advice: Take in divided doses, 2 to 4 times daily (exact times not critical).

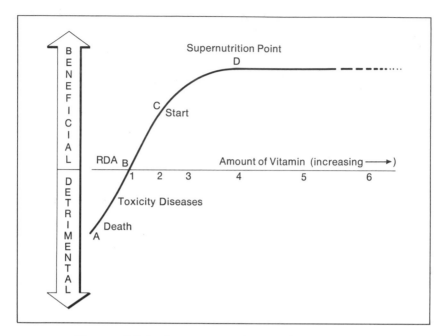

Figure A9.3 Supernutrition Curve: Vitamin B₂

Typical Values
Points   *Values*
1.   RDA is 1.8 mg.
2.   Supernutrition starting
            point is 10–25 mg.
3.   50 mg.
4.   100 mg.
5.   Does not apply.
6.   Does not apply.

Vitamin B₃ (Niacin, Niacinamide, Nicotinamide, Nicotinic Acid)

Vitamin B₃ exists in two main forms, niacin (or nicotinic acid) and niacinamide (or nicotinamide). The niacin form produces a "flushing" and itching of the skin. Although this condition is temporary and occurs only when niacin is first taken in higher doses, most people find it objectionable. Good sources are nut butters, meat, liver, fish, poultry, eggs, and whole-grain breads and cereals.

Agreed function: Vitamin B₃ is related to protein and carbohydrate metabolism.

Speculative function: To facilitate the cure of mental disturbances by correcting certain enzyme deficiencies.

Deficiency signs: Loss of appetite, nervousness, mental depression, soreness and redness of the tongue and skin

Figure A9.4 Supernutrition Curve: Vitamin B₃

Typical Values
Points	Values
1.	RDA is 20 mg.
2.	Supernutrition starting point is 50 mg.
3.	100 mg.
4.	250 mg-3 grams.
5.	Does not apply.
6.	Does not apply.

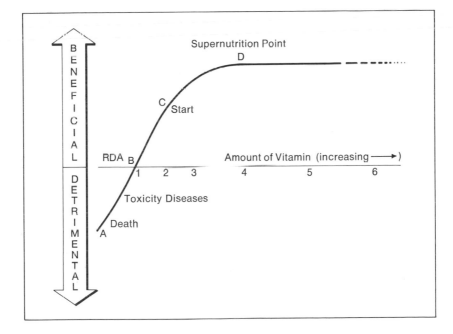

pigmentation, ulceration of the gums, and diarrhea. Gross deficiency results in pellagra.

Toxicity signs: None known.

Precautions: Be sure to include other B-complex vitamins with the Vitamin B₃. Reduce dosage if heart palpitations occur. Niacin causes skin flushing and sometimes itching when first taken in higher doses—niacinamide does not. Use with caution if you have glaucoma, severe diabetes, impaired liver function, or peptic ulcer.

Preferred forms: Niacinamide (or nicotinamide).

Dosage advice: Take in divided doses, 2 to 4 times daily (exact times not critical).

Vitamin B₅ (Pantothenic Acid)

Pantothenic acid is a water-soluble member of the vitamin B complex. Good sources are whole-grain cereals, legumes, and animal tissues.

Agreed function: Pantothenic acid is involved in adrenal gland function and is required to fight stress.

Speculative function: To correct certain enzyme deficiencies and improve mental processes. To help cure arthritis.

Deficiency signs: Headache, fatigue, muscle cramps, and reduced coordination.

Toxicity signs: None known.

Precautions: Be sure to include other B-complex vitamins with pantothenic acid.

Preferred form: Calcium panthothenate or pantothenic acid.

Dosage advice: Take in divided doses, 2 to 4 times daily (exact times not critical).

Vitamin B₆ (Pyridoxine, Pyridoxol, Pyridoxal, Pyridoxamine)

Vitamin B₆ is a water-soluble member of the vitamin B complex. It exists in three forms and often occurs in nature as a mixture of these three forms. This family was originally called pyridoxine, but more recently has been called pyri-

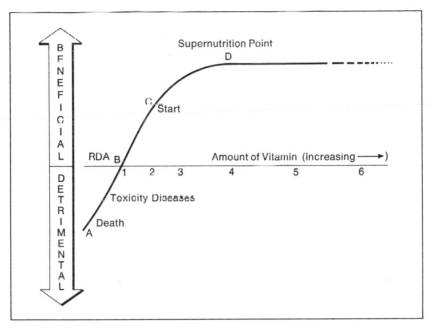

Figure A9.5 Supernutrition Curve: Vitamin B₅

Typical Values

Points	Values
1.	RDA is not given; a reasonable estimate would be 5–10 mg.
2.	Supernutrition starting point is 10–20 mg.
3.	25–50 mg.
4.	100 mg.
5.	Does not apply.
6.	Does not apply.

doxol—currently biochemists favor the term pyridoxol while nutritionists favor the term pyridoxine. The three forms of vitamin B₆ are pyridoxal, pyridoxol, and pyridoxamine. Good sources are liver, ham, lima beans, and corn.

Agreed function: Vitamin B₆ is involved in protein, fat, and sugar metabolism and is intimately concerned with the metabolism of the central nervous system.

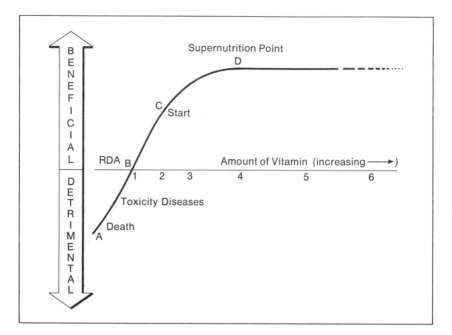

Figure A9.6 Supernutrition Curve: Vitamin B₆

Typical Values

Points	Values
1.	RDA is 2 mg.
2.	Supernutrition starting point is 10–25 mg.
3.	50 mg.
4.	100 mg.
5.	~~Does not apply.~~
6.	Does not apply.

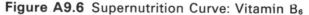

Speculative function: The utilization of vitamin B₆ in the coenzymes used to make lecithin in the body and convert cholesterol to cholesterol ester may make vitamin B₆ important in preventing heart disease. It also helps cure arthritis.

Deficiency signs: Loss of appetite, diarrhea, skin and mouth disorders, blindness.

Toxicity signs: None known (may turn urine yellow but this is normal).

Precautions: Be sure to include other B-complex vitamins with vitamin B₆. Reduce dosage if heart palpitations occur.

Preferred forms: None.

Dosage advice: Take in divided doses, 2 to 4 times daily (exact times not critical).

Vitamin B₁₂ (Cyanocobalamin)

Vitamin B₁₂ is a water-soluble member of the vitamin B complex. Requirements are in the microgram range, which is lower than the milligram range of the other B vitamins. Good sources are animal tissues, which can create a problem for vegetarians.

Agreed function: Vitamin B₁₂ is involved in the production of red blood cells and is usually known as the anti-anemia vitamin.

Speculative function: May be involved in nucleic-acid utilization and thus related to nucleic-acid therapy and aging.

Deficiency signs: Anemia and degeneration of the nervous system.

Toxicity signs: None known.

Precautions: Be sure to include other B-complex vitamins with vitamin B₁₂. Reduce dosage if heart palpitations occur.

Preferred forms: None.

Dosage advice: Take in divided doses, 2 to 4 times daily (exact times not critical).

Other Important Members of the Vitamin B Complex

Five members of the vitamin B complex (biotin, inositol, folic acid, PABA, and choline) are often overlooked. They can be considered minor members of the family only because they are often omitted from the less expensive formulations. Human needs for them are just as great as needs for any other vitamin. Often these minor B-complex vitamins are in commercially short supply. Biotin and inositol are acutely scarce, although it is hoped that the supply will appreciably increase by 1980. Good natural sources of this group are liver, yeast, eggs, and whole grains (the same as the major members of the vitamin B complex).

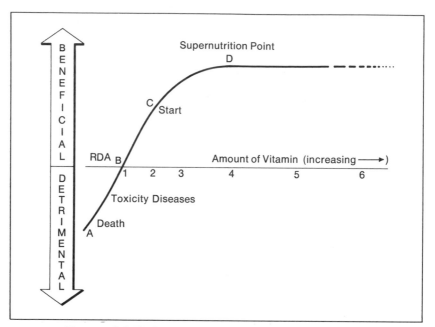

Figure A9.7 Supernutrition Curve: Vitamin B₁₂

Typical Values

Points	Values
1.	RDA is 3 mcg.
2.	Supernutrition starting point is 5–10 mcg.
3.	75 mcg.
4.	100 mcg.
5.	Does not apply.
6.	Does not apply.

Biotin

Biotin is essential to cellular metabolism, as it plays an important coenzyme role in the metabolism of fats, carbohydrates, and proteins. Biotin deficiency leads to anemia, muscular pain, and skin disorders. Early indications from experimental studies lead to speculation that a biotin deficiency may be involved in heart disease.

Small concentrations of biotin are found in all animal and

plant tissue, but good sources of biotin are eggs, liver, yeast, and kidney. Biotin is normally synthesized in large quantities by our own intestinal bacteria. Some drugs, such as antibiotics, can temporarily destroy these helpful bacteria, and some people may have intestinal conditions that inhibit this natural production of biotin.

Vitamin formulations vary markedly in biotin content. Often they change as the availability of biotin varies. Typically, a good multivitamin formulation may contain 2 to 50 mcg of biotin, a good B-complex formula may contain 10 to 50 mcg and a "super" B-complex 10 to 75 mcg. There is no known toxicity. It is estimated that a healthy person eating a balanced diet makes and ingests a total of 150 to 300 micrograms daily. Normal production and ingestion from foods overwhelm the minute amount available in vitamin pills. Personally, I use the biotin content of pills to judge the completeness of the formula.

Inositol

The precise role of inositol is unknown. Animals deficient in inositol grow poorly and show hair loss. No human vitamin function is yet claimed for inositol, thus the FDA does not recognize it as an essential vitamin. You may, however, remember that the FDA did not recognize vitamin E as an essential vitamin until 1957.

Inositol occurs naturally in fruits and cereals. Good sources are yeast, citrus fruits, wheat germ, lima beans, peas, and organ meats. It is possible, though not certain, that we may synthesize some inositol with the aid of our intestinal bacteria. Good vitamin formulations typically contain 10 to 500 mg of inositol in multivitamins and 50 to 1000 mg in B-complex formulations—if they contain any.

Folic Acid

Folic acid is really a family of several complex chemicals, but is generally referred to as one substance. It is present in all green-leafed vegetables, eggs, liver, kidney, wheat germ, and yeast. Folic acid is limited by the FDA to 0.4 mg per pill for adults and children over four years of age. Exceptions are pills specifically labeled for pregnant or lactating women, which may contain 0.8 mg each, and pills limited to prescription sales, which may contain 1.0 mg each. The FDA limits are applied not because of possible toxicity or any real danger, but solely to allow simpler diagnoses of pernicious anemia—when vitamin B_{12} is deficient, but folic acid is present in adequate amounts, pernicious anemia develops without its normal telltale signs in the blood cells. Thus the disease develops but can't be detected until it is too late to prevent irreversible damage. The FDA reasons that if B_{12} is deficient because of faulty assimilation by the body, this deficiency might be masked by the folic acid in vitamin pills. But then what about the folic acid in a regular diet?

The exact human daily requirement for folic acid is not known, but it is probably in the 0.1 to 2.0 mg range. There is no known toxicity.

PABA

Para-aminobenzoic acid (p-aminobenzoic acid or PABA) is an important growth factor for many microorganisms and a deficiency causes a loss of hair color in mice. However, no vitamin function has been shown in man, thus PABA is not yet recognized as an essential vitamin by the FDA. PABA is known in gerontology as an effective sun-screen to prevent skin-wrinkling and sunburn. In humans it has often restored gray hair to its normal color, but perhaps only in cases where graying was because of a vitamin B complex deficiency in the first place.

It is used by green-leafed vegetables to synthesize folic acid. As it is a part of folic acid, it can be found wherever folic acid occurs naturally. The best sources of PABA are liver, yeast, and rice. Vitamin pills typically contain 10 to 50 mg. There is no known toxicity.

Choline

By definition, choline is not a vitamin. It is a nutritionally important accessory food substance that for want of a better classification is grouped with the vitamins. It is widely found in nature, with high levels in animal tissues and lower levels in vegetables and cereals. The best source of choline is eggs. Choline may be useful in protecting our livers, kidneys, and arteries.

The actual need for choline may be only 10 to 20 mg per day, but several hundred milligrams have to be eaten to supply the body with 10 mg; most ingested choline is destroyed by the intestinal bacteria. "Normal" balanced diets contain 300 to 1000 mg of choline; multivitamin pills contain 20 to 500 mg if they contain any, and vitamin B complex formulas contain 50 to 100 mg. There is no known toxicity.

Biotin, choline, folic acid, inositol, and PABA are all safe in large quantities and are involved in protection against heart disease and stress. Several experiments have shown success in restoring natural hair coloring to those prematurely gray because of deficiencies in these vitamins—get as much of each as you can. A good B-complex formulation, liver, and yeast are your best sources.

Vitamin C (Ascorbic Acid)

Vitamin C is a water-soluble vitamin with no known toxicity. It is looked upon by some researchers as being more than a vitamin, as being actually a liver metabolite missing in humans as a result of a genetic accident. Good sources are citrus fruits, tomatoes, strawberries, cranberries, potatoes, and raw greens.

Agreed function: Vitamin C is necessary for the formation and renewal of the intercellular ground (or cement) substances which hold together the cells of all tissues, including bones, teeth, skin, organs, and capillary walls. Vitamin C detoxifies many poisonous substances, is important in healing processes and red blood formation, and is needed by the adrenal gland to fight stress.

Speculative function: Vitamin C has shown evidence of reducing the severity of cold symptoms. Several researchers claim evidence that vitamin C has antiviral and antibacterial properties. Vitamin C has been shown to reduce cholesterol deposits, and may help prevent cancer.

Deficiency signs: Bleeding and receding gums, unexplained bruises, slow healing, and scurvy.

Toxicity signs: None known (often increases the frequency of urination, but this is a harmless natural sign).

Figure A9.8 Supernutrition Curve: Vitamin C

Typical values

Points	Values
1.	RDA is 45 mg.
2.	Supernutrition starting point is 500–750 mg.
3.	2 g. (2,000 mg.).
4.	4 g.
5.	Does not apply.
6.	Does not apply.

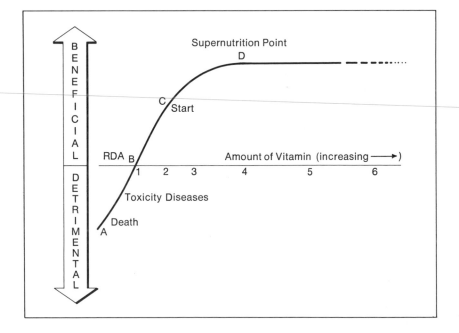

Precautions: Cut back dosage if diarrhea occurs. The sodium ascorbate form (often found in chewable tablets) should not be taken by people on low-salt (low-sodium) diets. People taking anticoagulants should consult their doctors. Vitamin C is a mild diuretic, but this is not a significant problem.

Preferred forms: (1) calcium ascorbate, the form in which it is stored in glands (not widely available); (2) ascorbic acid; (3) sodium ascorbate (not to be taken by people on low-salt diets); (4) rose hips, or other completely natural forms, make large doses impractical because of problems with sizes or amounts of pills.

Dosage advice: Take in divided doses, 2 to 4 times daily (exact times not critical). It is helpful to take milk or calcium tablets along with vitamin C. Many people claim better results when taking naturally occurring cofactors along with vitamin C; some, for example, prefer to drink natural citrus-fruit juice along with it. Be sure to take adequate vitamin B_{12}.

Vitamin D (Calciferol)

Vitamin D is present in nature in several forms, all of which occur only in animals. Provitamins D from vegetables can be converted in the body to vitamin D by the action of sunlight on the skin. Vitamin D is a fat-soluble vitamin with known toxicity. The two most common forms of vitamin D are vitamin D_2 (ergocalciferol or irradiated ergosterol) and vitamin D_3 (cholecalciferol). Good sources are sunlight and fish-liver oils.

Agreed function: Vitamin D is needed most during periods of growth for good bones and teeth. It is required throughout a person's life for calcium metabolism.

Deficiency signs: Weight loss, loss of appetite, cramps, poor bone formation, and rickets.

Toxicity signs: Unusual thirst, urinary urgency, vomiting, and diarrhea.

Precautions: People with heart disorders or kidney disease should use vitamin D with caution; everyone should be aware of its possible toxicity.

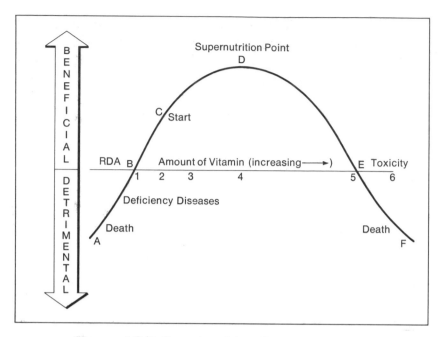

Figure A9.9 Supernutrition Curve: Vitamin D

Typical Values

Points	Values
1.	RDA is 400 IU.
2.	Supernutrition starting point is 400–500 IU.
3.	800 IU.
4.	1,000 IU.
5.	40,000 IU (2,000 IU in children).
6.	300,000 IU.

Preferred forms: (1) irradiated ergosterol (ergocalciferol); (2) fish oils; (3) others.

Dosage advice: Best absorbed if taken with meals.

Vitamin E (Tocopherol)

Vitamin E activity is possessed by a family of chemicals called tocopherols. The prime member is alpha-tocopherol, and lesser members of the family are the beta-, gamma-, and delta-tocopherols. Other related natural tocopherols have not shown significant vitamin E activity. Vitamin E is a fat-soluble vitamin and hence viewed as potentially toxic, but no signs of toxicity have been observed even in those who have taken high dosages over several decades. Good sources are whole grains, wheat germ, nuts, legumes, eggs, and sprouts.

Agreed function: Vitamin E is vital to normal reproduction.

Speculative function: A number of researchers see evidence to support claims that vitamin E slows the aging process, prevents heart disease, and reduces the incidence of cancer.

Deficiency signs: Discolored pigmentation, anemia. Other signs have been seen in animals, such as nutritional muscular dystrophy, testicle shrinkage, blood-vessel disorders, etc.

Toxicity signs: None known. Studies with growing chickens have shown growth abnormalities at very high dosages. One physician has reported increased fatigue associated with initiation of vitamin E therapy. If fatigue develops, check the creatine level monitored as part of your periodic blood analysis.

Precautions: People with overactive thyroids, diabetes, high blood pressure, or rheumatic hearts should proceed cautiously; start at 30 IU for a month, then increase by 30 IU each month until a tolerance limit is reached.

Preferred forms: (1) mixed tocopherols; (2) D-alpha-tocopheryl succinate or D-alpha-tocopheryl acetate; (3) DL-alpha-tocopheryl acetate or DL-alpha-tocopheryl succinate.

Dosage advice: Best absorbed if taken with meals or wheat-germ oil (one teaspoonful or 2 to 3 capsules, each 3 minims or more in size, of wheat-germ oil is adequate for this purpose). Try to take at times when you are not taking pills containing iron. Although the action of iron on vitamin E has been overemphasized, "free" iron in the same pill with vitamin E can destroy it. Chelated iron or strongly bound organic forms of iron will not attack vitamin E and the iron in food is usually chelated.

To double the blood content level of vitamin E, the dosage must be increased 40 times. Compared with the 100 IU level, a 500 IU level of vitamin E increases the blood level of vitamin E by only 9 percent.

Figure A9.10 Supernutrition Curve: Vitamin E

Typical Values

Points	Values
1.	RDA is 15 IU.
2.	Supernutrition starting point is 200 IU.
3.	400 IU.
4.	800 IU.
5.	No known toxicity.
6.	No known toxicity.

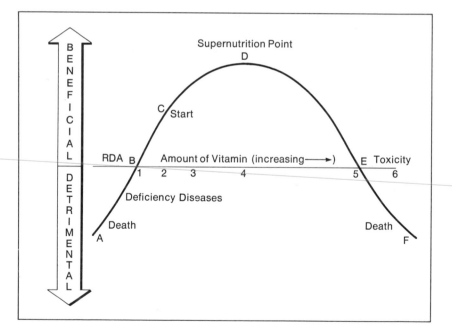

Appendix Ten
Selected References for the Monoclonal-Proliferation Explanation of Atherosclerosis

1. Moss, N.S., and Benditt, E.P. (1970) *Laboratory Investigation* 23, 231–245.
2. Moss, N.S., and Benditt, E.P. (1970) *Laboratory Investigation* 23, 521–535.
3. Poole, J.C.F., Cromwell, S.B., and Benditt, E.P. (1971) *American Journal of Pathology* 62, 391–404.
4. Schwartz, S.M., and Benditt, E.P. (1973) *Laboratory Investigation* 28, 699–701.
5. Benditt, E.P., and Benditt, J.M. (1973) *Proceedings of the National Academy of Science* 70, 1753–1756.
6. Ross, R., and Glomset, J.A. (1973) *Science* 180, 1332–1340.
7. Moss, N.S., and Benditt, E.P. (1974) *Federation Proceedings* 33, 624.
8. Vracko, R., and Benditt, E.P. (1974) *American Journal of Pathology* 75, 204–207.
9. Pearson, T.A., Wang, A., Solez, K., and Heptinstall, R.H. (1975) *American Journal of Pathology* 81, 379–387.
10. Article (1976) *Scientific News* 109, 260.
11. Kolata, Gina (1976) *Science* 194, 592–594.

Appendix Eleven
Frequently Asked Questions, Answered

Q. I have read time and time again that it's been proven that cholesterol and fats in food cause heart disease. Isn't that the case?

A. This is a common misconception. The opposite has been shown. Chapters 4 through 8 discuss the many tests that show that cholesterol and fats in food are not the culprits and in fact often show a protective effect because these foods are good sources of vitamins and minerals. The often misquoted Framingham study is a specific example.

Some improperly designed experiments did indicate such a relationship years ago, and since it's so easy to believe that food cholesterol is the villain because cholesterol is found in the plaques, authorities jumped the gun without proper confirmation. After decades of misinformation it's difficult for them to look at the newer evidence with an open mind.

Q. Why are we always reading that polyunsaturates are good for the heart or prevent heart disease?

A. Pure commercialism. These pseudo-drug ads designed to create cholesterolphobia create a market for newer, high-profit products such as margarines, egg-substitutes, meat-substitutes, low-fat dairy products, and the like.

Q. You say that low-cholesterol, low-fat diets do not affect heart disease, yet the Pritikin low-fat diet has had great success.

A. The Pritikin diet works because it is a low-calorie diet

well balanced in terms of micro-nutrients (vitamins and minerals). That it also happens to be a low-cholesterol, low-fat diet is incidental to its success. Another diet of the same calorie level and still as well-balanced in micro-nutrients would do just as well, whether it be low-carbohydrate, or whatever. Don't forget that exercise and nonsmoking play an important part in the Pritikin diet program.

Unfortunately, most low-cholesterol diets lack the nutrients necessary to prevent or cure heart disease. Most low-cholesterol diets have caused more damage than good. One specific example, explained in Chapter 7, is the excessively high level of polyunsaturates and the correspondingly low level of vitamin E available to protect the body against their damage.

Everybody will not do well on a low-fat diet. Many have done exceedingly well on Dr. Atkins' diet which is a high-fat diet. On this micronutrient-balanced diet, blood cholesterol levels drop and heart disease is arrested.

Q. I have read that low-cholesterol diets are helping reduce heart disease in Finland where people are heavy cholesterol eaters and have the world's highest rate of heart disease.

A. The misleading Finnish Mental Hospital study has often been written about by the low-cholesterol diet advocates. The first half of this study showed diet composition had no effect on heart disease, while the second half had a mix-up in diets in which the normal diet group received enough extra calories to put on an average of 40 pounds per patient. This serious flaw invalidates this portion of the experiment, but it is this portion that is so widely quoted by the low-cholesterol advocates. See Chapter 7 for a detailed discussion of this study.

Q. If vitamin E was effective against heart disease, why don't more doctors use it?

A. Doctors have had mixed opinions on vitamin E because there has not been an acceptable scientific explanation as to how vitamin E works against heart disease. The new evidence reported here shows that vitamin E prevents the blood from becoming sticky (as a result of platelet adhesion) and forming the clots that cause heart attacks. As doctors learn of these findings and try vitamin E in their practice, they will also become advocates. However they will have to learn to give vitamin E sufficient time to work on the blood platelets.

Q. Didn't a Canadian doctor find that vitamin E didn't help his heart patients?

A. Dr. T. W. Anderson evaluated vitamin E for use in heart disease and concluded that vitamin E was of no help. However, the length of time of the evaluation was insufficient for vitamin E to affect the blood-platelet adhesion as explained in Chapter 9. Long-term use relieves angina pain in more than 80 percent of heart patients and reduces the incidence of heart disease, as shown by my study. Others, including Drs. Wilfrid and Evan Shute, have found similar favorable results.

Q. Didn't a California doctor find that vitamin E made his patients feel tired?

A. Ninety-nine percent of the people taking vitamin E report increased energy. Of course it is possible that some people cannot tolerate vitamin E due to poor digestion or allergies. A very few people may have elevated creatine, which may produce a tired feeling. This small minority should cut back on dosage, but the advantage of heart attack protection for the general population shouldn't be lost because of some minor problem in a few people. There are other considerations before starting to take large doses of any vitamin. Chapter 9 discusses how to adjust the dose of vitamin E to your specific needs.

Q. If chelation therapy can save the lives of the thousands of people with inoperable heart disease, why don't more physicians use it? Is it safe?

A. It does save thousands of lives each year, and it is safe. The main objection was that the results were believed to be temporary. Studies show that the results last at least as long as those of bypass surgery and a significant advantage of chelation therapy is that follow-up treatment can be given at any time if blocking reoccurs. The dangers and pain of surgery discourage intervention until the very last minute.

Glossary

Alpha-tocopherol (α-tocopherol)	The principal form of vitamin E.
Angina pectoris	Chest pain due to insufficient oxygen for the heart's needs.
Antioxidant	A substance that prevents oxidation (reaction with oxygen) by sacrificing itself to the oxygen.
Anticoagulant	A substance that retards or prevents blood clots or coagulation.
Antithrombin	A specific type of anticoagulant.
Aorta	The largest artery in the body, through which blood leaves the heart.
Arrhythmia	An abnormal heartbeat rhythm.
Arteriosclerosis	The hardening of arteries that stiffens them and reduces their flexibility.
Atherogenic	Promoting atherosclerosis.
Atherosclerosis	The buildup of plaque in artery walls that narrows the artery opening.
Carcinogen	A substance that causes cancer.
Cardiovascular	Pertaining to the heart and blood vessels.
Cerebral hemorrhage	A broken or burst artery in the brain.
Chelation	The chemical complex formed between a mineral or metal having two positive charges and an organic compound that holds the mineral "in its structural claw."

Chelation therapy	A treatment that removes deposits from arteries with a chelating agent.
Cholesterol	A solid atomic alcohol produced in animals, including man, for their normal needs.
Cholesterolphobia	The needless and unfounded fear and avoidance of dietary cholesterol.
Cis fats	See discussion following *trans fats.*
Clonal	Pertaining to an identical duplicate, called a clone.
Collagen	The main structural protein of the body, making up about one-third of the total protein content.
Congestive heart failure	The inability of the heart to pump all of the blood returned to it.
Coronary occlusion	A blockage (clot) in a coronary artery that prevents blood from reaching the heart for its own use.
Coronary thrombosis	A clot in one of the branches of a coronary artery. A form of coronary occlusion often used synonymously with coronary occlusion.
Diastolic	The second number given in a blood-pressure measurement. The phase of greatest cardiac relaxation.
Dienes	Oxidized fragments of polyunsaturated fatty acids formed because of an antioxidant deficiency.
Diuretic	A substance that promotes the excretion of urine.
DNA	Deoxyribonucleic acid, the carrier of genetic information. The prime chemical of life and the only one that can reproduce itself.
EDTA	The chelating agent ethylene diamine tetra-acetic acid.

Electrocardiogram (EKG or ECG)	A graphic record of the electric currents produced by the heart.
Embolism	A blood clot obstructing a blood vessel.
Electrolyte	A substance that can conduct electricity when it is in solution.
Endarterectomy	Removal of material from within an artery.
Endothelium	The lining of a blood vessel.
Fibrillation	A disorganized, weak, and chaotic heart action (quiver).
Fibrin	A filamentous protein that forms to tangle blood cells and form a blood clot. It is formed by the action of thrombin on fibrinogen.
Fibrinogen	An enzyme in blood plasma which acts on thrombin (in the presence of calcium) to form fibrin to bring about the clotting of blood.
Free radicals	Highly reactive molecular fragments generally harmful to the body. A technical description is given in Appendix 3.
Free-radical scavenger	A substance that removes or inactivates a free radical.
Hypercholesterolemia	Elevated blood cholesterol.
Hyperlipidemia	Elevated blood fats.
Hyperlipoproteinemia	An abnormality in transporting blood fats that causes a genetic type of heart disease in a very small percetage of the population. See Appendix 2.
Hypertension	High blood pressure.
Infarct	The death of part of a tissue due to lack of blood.
Ischemia	The reduced blood supply to the heart due to atherosclerosis.
Intima	The innermost layer (but not the lining) of a blood vessel. See Figure 3.6 on page 33.

IU	International Unit. A standard unit of measure for many vitamins.
Lesion	A patch or plaque in a blood vessel. More accurately, any morbid change in or injury to tissue. Common usage uses the term interchangeably with plaque.
Lipid	A fat or fatty substance.
Lipid peroxidation	The rancifying or spoiling of fatty substances.
Lipoprotein	A simple protein conjugated with a fat that enables fat or fatlike compounds to be transported in the bloodstream (which is a water base).
Mcg	Microgram
Megavitamin	Large dose of a vitamin in comparison to the RDA.
Membrane	A layer that separates one part from another, such as the surface or "skin" of a cell, or the layer of tissue that lines a cavity.
Mg	Milligram
Microgram	Less than one ten-millionth of an ounce; more precisely, one-millionth of a gram or one-thousandth of a milligram.
Milligram	Less than one ten-thousandth of an ounce; more precisely, one-thousandth of a gram.
Monoclonal	Pertaining to the forming of many exact replicas of one parent cell.
Mutagen	A chemical that raises the rate of mutation above the spontaneous rate, thus causing abnormalities to increase.
Mutation	An abrupt change in a cell or organism.
Myocardial infarction	Damage to the heart because the blood supply has been cut off in a region of the heart muscle. A coronary.
Nucleic acid	A class of compounds found in cell nuclei. DNA and RNA are the most important nucleic acids.

Nucleoprotein	A class of protein in which molecules of a nucleic acid are conjugated (associated) with molecules of protein. Nucleoproteins are found in cell nuclei.
Nutrient	Any substance that nourishes the body, including vitamins, minerals, proteins, fats, and carbohydrates.
Pangamate	Vitamin B_{15}
Peripheral vascular disease	The reduction in blood supply to the smaller blood vessels.
Placebo	An inert pill used in controlled studies to simulate real medication.
Plaque	A patch or lesion in a blood vessel. Often described incorrectly as a deposit, but it is an eruption of cells from the middle layers of an artery through the wall into the artery interior (human). Plaques can continue to grow after they break through the artery wall.
Platelet	A round, disc-shaped blood cell, about half the size of a red blood cell, that plays an important role in clotting.
Platelet-adhesion index	A measurement of the stickiness of blood platelets.
Polyunsaturates	Soft or liquid fats having two or more structural locations capable of incorporating other atoms. Polyunsaturates are mostly of vegetable origin.
Proliferation	To reproduce or multiply, as in the reproduction of many daughter cells from a single cell.
P/S ratio	The ratio of polyunsaturated fats to saturated fats. If a diet contained 10 percent of its calories as polyunsaturates and 20 percent of its calories as saturates, the ratio would be 10 to 20 or a P/S of 10/20, or 0.5.
Radical	See "Free radical."

RDA	Recommended Daily Allowance of a vitamin or other nutrient. The Food and Nutrition Board of the National Research Council of the National Academy of Science (not a government organization, but a volunteer organization) makes judgments of daily nutrient intakes thought to be adequate for the maintenance of good nutrition in the population of the United States. These judgments are known as Recommended Dietary Allowances (RDA) and are value judgments based on the existing knowledge of nutritional science and are subject to revision as new knowledge becomes available. Many of the values established are controversial and reflect opinions of only one school of thought.
Saturates	Solid fats of animal origin. The fats are said to be saturated because their molecules will not take up any more hydrogen; thus their bonds are saturated.
Sphygmomanometer	An apparatus to measure blood pressure.
Stroke	A blockage of blood to a portion of the brain.
Systolic	The first number given in blood-pressure measurements. It pertains to the heart cycle in which the heart is in contraction.
Tachycardia	A very rapid heartbeat.
Thrombin	A substance in blood that combines with fibrinogen to form the fibrin needed to clot blood.
Thrombosis	The formation of a blood clot in the circulating blood. When it becomes detached from its original site, it is called a thrombotic embolus.
Tocopherol	Vitamin E

Trans fats	Fatty acids have a three-dimensional shape. *Cis* and *trans* refer to the spatial arrangement about the unsaturated multiple bond of the fatty acid. The natural form is *cis,* but during the refining of vegetable oils the spatial configuration of almost half the fatty acids is converted to the *trans* form. Additionally, during the manufacturing of margarine, hydrogen is added to make the oils solids (and more durable). During hydrogenation, about half of multiple bonds yield *trans* fats, which nature never does. The text gives quite a bit of information showing that the *trans* fats actually cause atherosclerosis. See Chapter 7 for details.
	The differences in hardness can be shown by comparing melting temperatures of the *cis* and *trans* forms. The *cis* form of oleic acid melts at 55° F, while the *trans* form melts at 111° F. The *cis* form of linoleic acid melts at 21° F, while the *trans* form melts at 82° F. See *Food For Nought* by Ross Hume Hall (Harper & Row, 1974) for further information.
Triglyceride	A fatty substance in the blood.
Uric acid	An acid in urine resulting from the breakdown of amino acids.
Unsaturates	A compound containing multiple bonds that are capable of adding hydrogen to the molecules, thus they are said to be unsaturated. If the molecule has more than one set of multiple bonds, it is said to be polyunsaturated. See "Polyunsaturates."
Vascular	Pertaining to blood vessels.

Suggested Readings

Cholesterol
The Cholesterol Controversy
Edward R. Pinckney, M.D., and Cathey Pinckney
Sherbourne Press, Inc., Los Angeles, 1973

Food for Nought
Ross Hume Hall
Harper & Row, N.Y., 1974

Supernutrition
Richard A. Passwater
The Dial Press, N.Y., 1975; Pocket Books, N.Y., 1976

Nutrition against Disease
Roger J. Williams
Pitman Publishing Co., N.Y., 1971

Vitamin E
The Complete, Updated Vitamin E Book
Wilfrid E. Shute, M.D.
Keats Publish. Co., New Canaan, Conn., 1975

Vitamin C
The Healing Factor
Irwin Stone
Grosset & Dunlap, N.Y., 1972

Vitamin C: The Powerhouse That Conquers More Than Just Colds.
Ruth Adams and Frank Murray
Larchmont Press, N.Y., 1972

Minerals
The Trace Elements and Man
H. A. Schroeder, M.D.
Devin-Adair Co., Old Greenwich, Conn., 1973

The Poisons Around Us
II. A. Schroeder, M.D.
Indiana University Press, Bloomington, 1974

Sugar
Low Blood Sugar and You
Carlton Fredericks, Ph.D., and Herman Goodman, M.D.
Constellation Int'l, N.Y., 1969

Nutrigenetics
Dr. R.O. Brennan with William C. Mulligan
M. Evans, N.Y., 1975

Psychodietetics
Dr. E. Cheraskin and Dr. W.M. Ringsdorf, with Arline
   Brecher
Stein and Day, N.Y., 1974

Megavitamin Therapy
Ruth Adams and Frank Murray
Larchmont Press, N.Y., 1973

Hypoglycemia
Dr. Charles Weller and B.R. Boyland
Award Books, N.Y., 1968

Sweet and Dangerous
John Yudkin, M.D.
Bantam Books, N.Y., 1973

Nutrition Periodicals
An important aid to maintaining optimum nutrition is a sub-
scription to a good nutrition magazine or newsletter. At
least once a month you will receive a reminder to watch
your diet and news of the latest discoveries in nutrition.
Among my favorites are the following:

Bestways
466 Foothill Blvd.
La Canada, Cal. 91011

Let's LIVE
444 Larchmont Blvd.
Los Angeles, Cal. 90004

National Health Federation Bulletin
212 W. Foothill Blvd.
Monrovia, Cal. 91016

Prevention
Rodale Press
Emmaus, Pa. 18049

Healthline
P.O. Drawer, S.E. Station
Washington, D.C. 20024

Healthview Newsletter
2677 State Highway 70
Manasquan, N.J. 08736

Index

Pooling Project and, 53–54; production of, 1, 6, 36, 37, 39, 46–47; as risk factor, 41
Cholesterolphobia, 4, 47
Cholestyramine, 89
Choline: dosage, 302, 353; function of, 336, 353; lecithin and, 157–158; sources of, 336, 349, 353
Christiansen, Jens, 309
Chromium, 152–153, 163–164, 337
Cigarette smoking: age and, 196, 197; arteries and, 198, 200, 202; blood clots and, 198; cadmium and, 151, 200, 202, 203; cholesterol-producing process and, 39; circulation and, 198–199; DNA mutation and, 6; exercise and, 205; heart attacks and, 9, 195, 196; high blood pressure and, 182, 200; increase in, 197, 200; life expectancy and, 195–196, 200–201; men and, 195, 196, 197; nonsmokers and, 201–205; oxygen starvation and, 199; quitting, 206–213; as risk factor, 3, 23, 41; stress and, 246; in Total Protection Plan, 2, 7, 278, 310; vitamin A and, 204–205; vitamin B₁₅ (pangamate) and, 203–204; vitamin C and, 131, 204; vitamin E and, 201, 203; women and, 18, 196, 197, 200–201
Circulation: cigarette smoking and, 198–199; magnesium and, 141; vitamin B₁₅ (pangamate) and, 124
Cis-fatty acids, 87
Citrus fruits, 336, 351, 353
Clams, 337
Clarke, Norman, 253, 260, 263
Clofibrate, 89, 90–92, 100
Coconut oil, 81
Cofactor, 125–126
Collagen, 6, 32, 36

Congenital defects, 9, 11, 24–25
Connors, W. E., 83
Cooper, Theodore, 172–173
Copper, 150–152, 302, 304
Corday, Eliot, 256
Corn, 118, 170, 337, 347
Corn grits, 125
Corn oil, 21, 69, 76, 81, 84, 85, 87, 88
Cornstock, George W., 212–213
Coronaries. See Heart attacks
Coronary bypass operation, 248–249, 255–257, 260
Coronary Drug Project Research Group, 90–92
Coronary heart disease, 26. See also Heart disease
Coronary sclerosis, 121
Coronary thrombosis: death from, 11–13, 15–19, 21, 22; defined, 11; epidemic nature of, 9–19, 22; first reporting of, 14; major pathway to, 42; men and, 9, 13, 17–19; modern life style and, 23; reducing chances of, 23; symptoms of, 13; vitamin C deficiency and, 133; women and, 13, 17, 19; younger age groups and, 15, 17, 18
Corrigan, J. J., 100
Cottonseed oil, 81
Craig, Marjorie, 236
Cranberries, 353
Crawford, Margaret D., 142, 146, 147
Crawford, T., 142
Creatine, 362
Creech, B. G., 49
Cromwell, S. B., 34
Crude fiber (CF), 169–170
Cryer, Phillip, 199
Cyanocobalamin. See Vitamin B₁₂
Cysteine, 205, 262–263

Dahl, Lewis K., 243–244
Dalderup, L. M., 166